U0333882

医学口袋书系列

实用手术室
专业英语会话

名誉主编	汪　晖		
主　　编	陈　红	曾铁英	
副 主 编	李　岩	吴　波	
编　　者	周秀娟	邹　康	陈梦妮
	王　荃	余云红	黎湘艳
	李　乔		

华中科技大学出版社
http://www.hustp.com
中国·武汉

内 容 简 介

本书分两部分,第一部分为专业词汇与短语,第二部分为手术室实用会话。本书针对不同场景提供较全的沟通用语,以便读者举一反三,将各部分所学对话与专业术语进行融合推广应用到其他类似情境之中。本书可用作指导新护士上岗和护理专业学生学习,也可用作护理临床、科研和教学人士参考。

图书在版编目(CIP)数据

实用手术室专业英语会话/陈红,曾铁英主编.—武汉:华中科技大学出版社,2020.6
ISBN 978-7-5680-5990-9

Ⅰ.①实… Ⅱ.①陈… ②曾… Ⅲ.①手术室-英语-口语 Ⅳ.①R197.38

中国版本图书馆 CIP 数据核字(2020)第 023072 号

实用手术室专业英语会话　　　陈　红　曾铁英　主编
Shiyong Shoushishi Zhuanye Yingyu Huihua

策划编辑:周芬娜	责任校对:李　琴
责任编辑:李　昊	责任监印:徐　露
封面设计:刘　婷	

出版发行:华中科技大学出版社(中国·武汉)　　电话:(027)81321913
　　　　　武汉市东湖新技术开发区华工科技园　邮编:430223

录　　排:华中科技大学惠友文印中心
印　　刷:武汉科源印刷设计有限公司
开　　本:880mm×1230mm　1/32
印　　张:5.5　插页:2
字　　数:159千字
版　　次:2020年6月第1版第1次印刷
定　　价:36.00元

前　言

　　进入 21 世纪以来,随着经济、文化全球化的加速发展,各国之间的交流与沟通越来越频繁,越来越多的国际友人来到中国学习、访问、定居,随之而来的外籍病人或外宾也日益增多;同时,随着我国护理事业的长足发展,越来越多优秀的中国护士走出国门,在国际护理舞台上展现自己的风采。为了给护理工作者尤其是手术室护理人员在临床上与国际友人交流、沟通时提供参考,同时,为了给手术室护士在国际舞台上展现手术室专业技能时提供有效的指导,编者经过两年的收集、整理资料,精心编撰了此书。

　　本书的特点主要是针对手术室的工作环境,提供在不同的场景下与外籍病人或者外宾交流时常用的英语会话以及手术室护士在配合外籍手术医生进行手术时常用的英语会话。目前市面出现较多的医务英语类书籍主要是针对进入医院门诊就诊、检查身体、住院出院等环节,提供日常英语会话,但很少涉及手术室方面。因此通过本书,读者会进一步了解在这方面与患者或外籍学者交流的方式。

　　全书分为两大部分,第一部分为专业词汇,包括手术室护理相关专业术语、常用操作技术、常用称谓、医疗仪器与设备、常用医疗器材以及手术名称;第二部分为手术室常用英文例句,针对不同场景如术前等待间、

I

术前准备、术中配合、术后苏醒与交接、术后回访等,提供了较全的沟通用语,充分体现了"关爱生命,以人为本,以德施护"的人本护理观。除此之外,它还包括不同专科手术配合时常用的套句,便于读者通过反复训练,牢记常用句型,在不同的语境中准确地脱口而出。

　　本书所选语句都是手术室工作环境中护理的常用语,内容丰富、新颖,语言简洁,可用于指导新护士上岗和护理专业学生学习,也可作为护理临床、科研和教学人士参考。全书编写历经两年时间,全体参编人员付出了艰辛的劳动,后经过华中科技大学同济医学院附属同济医院护理部汪晖主任、曾铁英副主任等老师的精心雕琢,得以成型,谨对上述领导、同仁致以衷心的谢意。由于编者水平有限,难免有疏漏和不当之处,敬请广大读者、专家和护理同仁批评、指正,在此深表感谢!

编者
2020 年 4 月

目　录

第一部分　专业词汇

目　录

实用手术室专业英语会话

六、**Names of surgeries**

目录

第二部分　手术室常用英文例句

一、**Common communication sentences**

目

录

实用手术室专业英语会话

第一部分

专业词汇

一、Professional terms for operating nursing
手术室护理相关专业术语

1. nursing terminology
护理名词

nursing process

护理程序

nursing assessment

护理评估

nursing planning

护理计划

nursing diagnosis

护理诊断

nursing evaluation

护理评价

nursing intervention

护理措施

daily care of the patient

病人日常护理

morning（evening）care

晨（晚）间护理

oral hygiene（mouth care）

口腔卫生（口腔护理）

bed making

整理床铺

flossing the teeth

清洁牙垢

brushing the teeth

刷牙

bathing

洗澡

dentures care

清洗假牙

perineal care

清洗会阴

cleanliness

清洁

care of nails and feet

指甲修剪和洗脚

massage

按摩

changing hospital gowns

更换住院服装

bedsore care

压伤护理

2. nursing operation
护理操作

cardiac catheterization

心导管插入

catheterization

导管插入

urethral catheterization

导尿术

decompression

减压

cerebral decompression

脑减压

orbital decompression

眼眶减压

decompression of spinal cord

脊髓减压

decompression of rectum

直肠减压

gastro-intestinal decompression

胃肠减压

dialysis

透析

peritoneal dialysis

腹膜透析

hemodialysis

血液透析

drainage

引流、导液

open drainage

开放引流法

closed drainage

密闭引流法

vaginal drainage

阴道引流法

postural drainage

体位引流法

aspiration（suction）drainage

吸引导液（引流）

negative pressure drainage

负压吸引法

suctioning

吸引引流

upper airway suctioning

上呼吸道抽吸法

wound suctioning

伤口吸引

nasogastric suctioning

鼻胃抽吸

blind enema

肛管排气法

enema

灌肠

glycerin enema

甘油灌肠

barium enema

钡灌肠

turpentine enema

松节油灌肠

magnesium sulfate enema

硫酸镁灌肠

soapsuds enema

肥皂水灌肠

retention (non-retention) enema

保留(无保留)灌肠

feeding

喂养

nasal feeding

鼻饲法

rectal feeding

直肠营养法

heat/cold applications

冷、热敷

applying cold compresses

冷敷

applying hot compresses

热敷

injection

注射

applying hot soaks

湿热敷

intracutaneous injection

皮内注射

hypodermic injection

皮下注射

intramuscular injection

肌肉注射

intraocular injection

眼球注射

subconjunctival injection

结膜下注射

nasal injection

鼻内注射

intrapleural injection

胸膜腔注射

peritoneal injection

腹膜腔注射

intrauterine injection

子宫内注射

rectal injection

直肠注射

irrigation

冲洗

bladder irrigation

膀胱冲洗

vaginal irrigation

阴道冲洗

lavage

灌洗

pleural lavage

胸膜腔灌洗

peritoneal lavage

腹膜腔灌洗

gastric lavage

洗胃

intestinal lavage

洗肠

isolation

隔离、分离

contact isolation

接触隔离

strict isolation

严密隔离

protective isolation

保护性隔离

vaginal medication

阴道给药法

venous transfusion

静脉输血

blood transfusion

输血

plasma transfusion

输血浆

serum transfusion

输血清

measurement of vital signs

测量生命体征

taking a radial pulse

测量桡动脉脉搏

counting respirations

计呼吸次数

measuring blood pressure

测量血压

taking oral（rectal，axillary）temperature

量口腔（直肠、腋下）体温

giving a cold（an alcohol）sponge bath

冷水（酒精）擦浴

assisting the patient to take a sit bath

帮病人坐浴

emergency care（first aid）

急救护理（急救）

cardiopulmonary resuscitation

心肺复苏术

mouth-to-mouth resuscitation

口对口人工呼吸

emergency care for fainting（shock，stroke）victims

昏厥（休克、中风）患者急救

emergency care used to control hemorrhage

止血急救

emergency care given to help a patient who is vomiting

呕吐患者急救

emergency care for a patient during a seizure

癫痫发作急救

hospice care

临终护理

3. diet nursing
饮食护理

absolute diet（fasting）

禁食

smooth（soft）diet

细软饮食

balanced diet

均衡饮食

diabetic diet

糖尿病饮食

fat-free diet

无脂饮食

salt-free diet

无盐饮食

full diet

全食，普通饮食

high caloric diet

高热量饮食

high-carbohydrate diet

高糖类饮食

high-protein（protein rich）diet

高蛋白（富含蛋白质）饮食

light diet

易消化饮食

liquid diet

流质饮食

high fat diet

高脂饮食

low fat diet

低脂饮食

low caloric diet

低热量饮食

low-protein diet

低蛋白饮食

low-residue diet

低渣饮食

regimen diet

规定食谱

二、Operation terms for operating room

手术室常用操作技术

1. disinfection and sterilization
消毒灭菌

asepsis

无菌（法）

integral asepsis

完全无菌

cleaning

清洁

disinfection

消毒

autoclaving

高压蒸汽消毒

autoclave sterilizer

高压蒸汽灭菌器

steam sterilizer

蒸汽灭菌器

soaking

浸泡

disinfectant

消毒剂

sterile field

无菌区

sterile pack

无菌包

terminal disinfection

终末消毒

sterilization

灭菌、消毒

disinfection by ultraviolet light

紫外线消毒

chemical sterilization

化学灭菌法

contact isolation

接触隔离

protective isolation

保护性隔离

2. preparing the patient for the surgery
手术准备

preoperative shaving

术前备皮

postoperative care

术后护理

applying elastic stockings

穿弹力袜

applying elastic bandages

用弹性绷带

coughing and deep-breathing exercises

咳嗽呼吸练习

3. posture placement
体位安置

fowler's position

半坐卧位

supine position

仰卧位

horizontal position

平卧位

lateral position

侧卧位

prone position

俯卧位

lithotomy position

截石位

thyroid position

甲状腺体位

sitting position

坐位

anterior

前的

posterior

后的

superior

上的

inferior

下的

medial

中间的

lateral

侧边的

proximal

近端的

distal

远端的

superficial

浅表的

deep

深的

flexion

屈曲

extension

伸屈

rotation

旋转

inversion

内翻

eversion

外翻

abduction

外展

adduction

内收

elevation

上提

depression

下压

4. anesthetic intubate
麻醉插管

epidural anesthesia

硬膜外麻醉

intravenous anesthesia

静脉麻醉

combined anesthesia

复合麻醉

nerve block

神经阻滞

三、Names related to operating room
手术室常用称谓

1. medical title
医务人员名称

superintendent; director of the hospital

负责人;院长

controller

总务科长

director of administration

医务处主任

hospital departments

医院科室

specialist; expert

专家

doctors and nurses

医师和护士

head of ×× department

某科主任

chief physician

主任医师

associate chief physician

副主任医师

attending doctor

主治医师

resident doctor

住院医师

intern doctor

实习医生

clinician

临床医师

general practitioner

全科医师

specialist

专科医师

physician

内科医师

ophthalmologist

眼科医师

dentist

牙科医师

ENT doctor

耳鼻喉科医师

orthopedist

骨科医师

dermatologist

皮肤科医师

gynecologist

妇科医师

urologist surgeon

泌尿外科医师

anesthetist

麻醉科医师

neurosurgeon

神经外科医师

dietician

营养科医师

plastic surgeon

矫形外科医师

physiotherapist

理疗医师

obstetrician

产科医师

pediatrician

儿科医师

radiologist

放射科医师

midwife

助产士

head of the nursing department

护理部主任

chief head nurse

总护士长

supervisor nurse

科护士长

ward head nurse

病区护士长

night nursing supervisor

夜班总值班护士长

chief superintendent nurse

主任护师

supervisor nurse

主管护师

senior nurse

护师

primary nurse

责任护士

registered nurse

注册护士

circulating/utility nurse

巡回护士

scrub nurse

器械护士

assistant nurse

助理护士

associate nurse

辅助护士

nutrition nurse

营养护士

student nurse

实习护士

laboratory technician

化验员

registrar

挂号员

sanitation worker

消毒员

cleaner

清洁员

2. name of clinical department
临床科室名称

general hospital

综合医院

children's hospital

儿童医院

inpatient department

住院部

admission office

入院处

outpatient department

门诊部

emergency department

急诊科

ENT department

耳鼻喉科

department of pediatrics

儿科

department of orthopedics

骨科

medical department

内科

surgical department

外科

plastic surgery

整形外科

department of cardiology

心内科

department of anesthesia

麻醉科

department of radiology

放射科

registration office

挂号处

pharmacy/dispensary

药房

general ward

普通病房

isolation ward

隔离病房

infectious ward

传染病房

observation ward

观察病房

dressing room

包扎室

operating room

手术室

private/single ward

单人病房

preparation room

准备室

injection room

注射室

sterilizing room

灭菌室

therapeutic room

治疗室

recovery room

恢复室

isolation unit

隔离病房

hyperbaric oxygen chamber

高压氧舱

四、Common equipment in operating room

手术室常用设备

operating bed

手术床

operating lamp

手术灯

shadowless lamp

无影灯

anesthesia machine

麻醉机

laparoscope

腹腔镜

ultrasonic wave apparatus

超声波机

sphygmomanometer

血压计

nuclear magnetic resonance

核磁共振

electrocardiac monitor

心电监护仪

autoclave sterilizer

高压蒸气灭菌器

electrocardiograph

心电图机

computer tomography

(CT)计算机断层摄影

defibrillator

除颤仪

binocular microscope

双目显微镜

wall oxygen outlet

壁式输氧机

ventilator

呼吸机、呼吸器

automatic ventilator

自动呼吸机

positive pressure ventilator

正压呼吸机

negative pressure ventilator

负压呼吸机

bronchoscope

支气管镜

direct laryngoscope

直接喉镜

fiberoptic esophagscope

纤维食管镜

esophagoscope

食管镜

flexible bronchofiberscope

可弯性纤维支气管镜

gastrofiberscope

纤维胃镜

gastroscope

胃镜

colposcope

阴道镜

metroscope

子宫镜

head mirror

头镜

otoscope

耳镜

proctoscope

直肠镜

cystoscope

膀胱镜

ophthalmoscope

眼底镜

pacemaker

起搏器

nasal speculum

鼻窥器、鼻镜

speculum oris

张口器

urethral speculum

尿道窥器

rectal speculum

直肠窥镜,直肠张开器

vaginal speculum

阴道窥器

sputum suction apparatus

吸痰器

mechanical suction

机械吸吮器

wall suction

壁式引流器

oxygen inhalator

氧吸入器

stethoscope

听诊器

suction apparatus

吸引器

electric suction

电动吸引器

wheel chair

轮椅

alcohol burner

酒精灯

drying baker

干燥器

leg brace

腿支架

stretcher

担架

crutch

拐杖

bedside rails

床栏

ultraviolet lamp

紫外线灯

first-aid kit

急救箱

surgical isolator

外科手术消毒包

五、Medical equipment of operating room

手术室常用医疗器材

1. consumable materials in operating room

手术室耗材

operating coat/cap

手术衣/帽

gauze mask

口罩

sterile gloves

无菌手套

disposable glove

一次性手套

sutures

缝线

ribbon gut

肠线

absorbable suture

可吸收缝线

splint

夹板

mattress

床垫

absorbent cotton

脱脂棉

cotton balls

棉球

bandage

绷带

elastic bandage

弹力绷带

dressing

敷料

adhesive plaster

胶布

gauze

纱布

cotton sticks

棉签

petrolatum gauze

凡士林纱布

gelatin sponge

明胶海绵

swab

拭子、药签

syringe

注射器

hypodermic syringe

皮下注射器

trocar

套(管)针

needle

针头

barrel

筒、管

pump

筒、泵

funnel

漏斗

Murphy's drip bulb

墨菲滴管

dressing bowl/basin

换药碗/盆

ampule

安瓿

ice bag

冰袋

ice cap

冰帽

incubator

保温箱

kidney basin

弯盆

medicine cup

药杯

vial

小瓶、密封瓶

plunger

活塞

scales

磅秤

sand bag

沙袋

specimen container

取样器皿

specimen bottle

标本瓶

sucker

吸管

test tube

试管

thermometer

体温表

tourniquet

止血带

transfusion apparatus

输血器

tray

托盘

urine bag

尿袋

breast binder

裹胸带

binder

腹带、绷带

elbow protector

肘护套

sling

悬带

scrotal support

阴囊托

gastric tube

胃管

rectal tube

肛管

catheter

导管

flexible catheter

软导管

perfusion cannula

灌注导管

wash-out cannula

冲洗套管

three-channel tube

三腔管

double current (two-way) catheter

双腔导管

indwelling catheter

留置导尿管

female catheter

女用导尿管

suction tube

吸引管

cardiac catheter

心导管

dialyser

透析膜

prostatic catheter

前列腺导尿管

dialyzator

透析器

tracheal catheter

气管吸引导管

drainage-tube

引流管

elastic drainage-tube

橡皮引流管

glass drainage-tube

玻璃引导管

enemator

灌肠器

intubator

插管器

artificial blood vessel

人造血管

irrigator

冲洗器

dropper

滴管

spatula

压舌板

tracheal tube

气管套管

ancillary supplies

辅助用品

paddles/pads

电极板、电极片

oxygen face mask

氧气面罩

cuff

袖带

2. surgical instruments
手术器械

1) basic instruments

常用基本器械

blade handle/holder

手术刀柄

blade（scalpel）

手术刀片

operating scalpel/knife

手术刀

scissors

剪刀

forceps

钳子

dissecting forceps

解剖镊

vessel clamp

止血钳、血管夹

S form retractor

S 型拉钩

mosquito forceps

蚊式止血钳

needle holder

持针器

towel clip

布巾钳

allis

组织钳

toothed forceps

有齿镊

plain forceps

无齿镊

sponge holder(forceps)

海绵钳

tissue forceps

组织镊

gun shape forceps

枪状镊

hemostatic clamp

止血夹

double hook skin retractor

双爪皮拉钩

mouth gag

开口器

hook

拉钩、电钩

electric scalpel

电刀

bipolar coagulation forceps

双极电凝镊

scalp needle

头皮针

bulldog clamp

血管夹

2) surgical instruments for specialist

   专科手术器械

(1) ophthalmology

   眼科

chalazion forceps

霰粒肿镊

ciliary forceps

睫毛镊

conjunctival forceps

结膜镊

corneal forceps

角膜镊

iris forceps

虹膜镊

lachrymal sac forceps

泪囊镊

eyelid retractor

眼睑拉钩

small curved scissors

小弯剪

ophthalmostat

眼球固定器

iris scissors

虹膜剪

lacrimal probe

泪管探针

eye speculum

开睑器

sclerotic puncher

巩膜打孔器

small straight scissors

小直剪

iris replacer

虹膜复位器

vitrectomy device

玻璃体切除器

capsulotomy forceps

晶体破囊镊

vitreous cutter

玻璃体切割器

eversion forceps

倒睫镊

canaliculus dilator

泪点扩张器

squeezing forceps

砂眼压榨镊

strabismus retractor

斜视牵开器

(2) otorhinolaryngology
耳鼻喉科

tonsil scissors

扁桃剪

tonsillectome

扁桃体切除器

sprayer

喷雾器

tonsil dissector

扁桃体剥离器

cerumen hook

盯聍钩

tonsil seizing forceps

扁桃体夹持钳

geniculate tweezers

膝状镊

instruments for nasoantral centesis

鼻窦穿刺器械

nasoantral centesis needle

鼻上颌窦穿刺针

tonsil ligature forceps

扁桃体结扎钳

(3) stomatology

口腔科

oral lamp

口腔灯

tooth pick

牙签

dental pliers

牙钳

probe

探针

punch

钻孔器

cheek retractor

口角拉钩

stump elevator

牙残根梃子

dental engine

牙钻机

enamel cutter

牙釉凿刀

dentiscalprum

牙刮

tongue depressor

压舌板

airdent

气磨洞形器

oral airway

口腔导气管

antroscope

上颌窦镜

antrotome

窦刀

articulator

咬合架

bridgework

(牙)桥托

pharyngeal brush

咽刷

excavating bur

牙挖钻

dental burnisher

牙磨光器

mastoid curette

乳突刮匙

periodontal curette

牙周刮匙

teeth cushion

牙垫

tongue forceps

舌钳

tonsil hemostatic forceps

扁桃体止血钳

mouth saw

口内锯

pulp canal reamer

牙髓根管扩大器

double-ended dental scale

双头洁牙器

dental nerve canal plug

牙神经根管填充器

(4) general surgery
普外科

abdominal apparatus

腹部器械

biopsy forceps

活检钳

curette

刮匙

intestinal spatula

压肠板

intestinal clamp

肠钳

bile duct probe

胆道探子

lithotomy forceps

取石钳

kidney clamp

肾钳

grasper

抓钳

non-traumatic grasper

无损伤抓钳

Kocher forceps

可可钳

angle clamp

直角钳

babcock forceps

阑尾钳

lung grasping forceps

肺叶钳

abdominal retractor

腹部拉钩

thyroid retractor

甲状腺拉钩

skin retractor

皮肤拉钩

amputation retractor

截肢拉钩

scalp hemostat clip

头皮止血夹

scalp clip applying forceps

头皮夹钳

cranial drill

颅骨钻

wire saw

线锯

brain spatulas

脑压板

laminectomy rongeur

椎板咬骨钳

rib shear

肋骨剪

self-retaining brain retractor

脑自动撑开器

rib contractor

肋骨合拢器

ventricular puncture needle

脑室穿刺针

micro scissors

显微剪

wire scissors

钢丝剪

bone holding forceps

持骨钳

nucleus pulposus clamp

髓核钳

rongeur

咬骨钳

bone mallet

骨锤

bone knife

骨刀

periosteal elevator

骨膜分离器

bone chisel

骨凿

amputation saw

截肢锯

mastoid retractor

乳突撑开器

skin graft knife

植皮刀

lamina spreader

椎板撑开器

electronic bone drill

电动骨钻

vein stripper

静脉剥脱器

mitral valve dilator

二尖瓣瓣膜扩张器

insufflation needle

气腹针

(5) gynaecology and obstetrics
妇产科

vaginal speculum

窥阴器

uterine dilator

子宫扩张器

uterine sound

宫腔探针

cervical clamps

宫颈钳

uterine manipulator

举宫器

obstetric forceps

产钳

metal catheter

金属导尿管

uterine curette

子宫刮匙

detacher

剥离器

vaginal retractor

阴道牵开器

cervix dilator

子宫颈扩张器

六、Names of surgeries
手术名称

1. ophthalmology
眼科

aspiration of cataract

白内障吸出术

enucleation of eyeball

眼球摘除术

corneal grafting

角膜移植

correction of entropion

睑内翻矫正术

dacryocystectomy

泪囊摘除术

lacrimal canalicular anastomosis

泪小管吻合术

incision of hordeolum

麦粒肿切开术

operation of pterygium

翼状胬肉手术

goniopuncture

前房角穿刺术

gonioectomy

前房角切除术

keratotomy

角膜切开术

kerectomy

角膜切除术

sclerectomy

巩膜切除术

corneal suture，keratorhaphy

角膜缝合术

vitrectomy

玻璃体切除术

corneoscleral trephination

角巩膜环钻术

omentorrhaphy

网膜缝合术

cryoextration of cataract

白内障冷冻摘除术

omentectomy

网膜切除术

intraocular lens implantation

人工晶体植入术

trabeculectomy

小梁切除术

correction of squint

斜视矫正术

lens extraction

晶体摘除

extraction of intra-ocular foreign body

眼内异物摘除

irrigation and probing of lacrimal passages

泪道冲洗和探通术

2. otorhinolaryngology
耳鼻喉科

mastoidectomy

乳突切开术

nasal、paranasal tumors resection

鼻腔、鼻窦肿瘤切除术

otoplasty

耳成形术

closed reduction of nasal bone

鼻骨闭合复位

myringotomy

鼓膜切开术

excision of turbinates

鼻甲切除术

myringoplasty

鼓膜成形术

nasal polypectomy

鼻息肉切除术

tympanoplasty

鼓室成形术

septoplasty

（鼻）中隔成形术

tracheostomy

气管切开术

sinusotomy

鼻窦切开术

tonsillectomy

扁桃体切除术

submuscous resection of nasal septum

鼻中隔黏膜下切除术

tonsilloadenoidectomy

扁桃体腺样增殖体切除术

3. stomatology
   口腔科

filling

牙填充

dental prosthetics

镶牙

tooth extraction

拔牙

laryngectomy and laryngostomy

喉切除术和喉造口术

parotidectomy

腮腺切除术

orthodontic treatment

牙矫正术

repair of cleft palate

腭裂修补术

periodontal treatment

牙周治疗

excision of parotid tumor

腮腺肿瘤切除术

radical resection of parotid adenocarcinoma

腮腺癌根治术

partial glossectomy

舌部分切除术

maxillectomy

下颌骨切除术

excision of submaxillary gland

颌下腺切除术

radical neck dissection

颈淋巴结清扫术

4. neurosurgery
神经外科

suprasellar meningioma resection

鞍上脑膜瘤切除术

intraorbital tumors resection

眶内肿瘤切除术

pituitary adenoma resection

垂体腺瘤切除术

craniopharyngioma resection

颅咽管瘤切除术

optic pathway and hypothalamic glioma resection

视路和下丘脑胶质瘤切除术

sphenoid ridge meningioma resection

蝶骨嵴脑膜瘤切除术

tumors of the infratemporal fossa resection

颞下窝肿瘤切除术

acoustic neuroma resection

听神经瘤切除术

brain stem tumors resection

脑干肿瘤切除术

resection of arterial aneurysm

动脉瘤切除术

decompression

减压术

excision of brain tumor

脑瘤切除术

exploratory craniotomy

开颅探查术

removed of intracranial hematoma

颅内血肿清除术

repair of dura defect

硬脑膜缺损修补术

extraintracranial artery anastomosis

颅内外动脉吻合

5. cardiovascular surgery and thoracic surgery
心血管外科和胸外科

abdominal aortic and iliac artery bypass

腹主动脉—髂动脉搭桥术

endarterectomy of abdominal aorta

腹主动脉内膜剥脱术

embolectomy by arteriotomy

动脉切开取栓术

carotid body tumor resection

颈动脉体瘤切除术

abdominal aortic aneurysm resection

腹主动脉瘤切除术

hemangioma resection

血管瘤切除术

aortocoronary bypass

主动脉冠状动脉分流

dilation of aortic valular stenosis

主动脉瓣狭窄扩张术

heart transplantation

心脏移植

heart valve replacement

心脏瓣膜置换术

complete intracardiac repair of Fallot's Tetralogy

法洛完全修复术

ligation of patent ductus arteriosis

动脉导管未闭结扎术

repair of auricular septal defect

房间隔缺损修补术

repair of ventricular septal defect

室间隔缺损修补术

repair if valvular insufficiency

瓣膜闭锁不全的修补

pericardiectomy

心包切除术

peicardiotomy

心包切开术

pulmonary embolectomy

肺动脉栓子切除术

closed drainage of pleural cavity

胸腔闭式引流

exploratory thoracotomy

开胸探查

lobectomy of lungs

肺叶切除

local excision of tumor of lungs

肺肿瘤局部切除术

parial esophagectomy and reconstruction of esophagus

食管部分切除与重建

6. general surgery
普外科

thyroidectomy

甲状腺切除术

subtotal thyroidectomy

甲状腺次全切除术

thyroid lobectomy

甲状腺叶切除术

thyroid cancer radical resection

甲状腺癌根治性切除术

adenomammectomy

乳腺切除术

breast cancer extensive radical mastectomy

乳腺癌广泛根治切除术

breast cancer modified radical mastectomy

乳腺癌改良根治术

intraductal papilloma excision

导管内乳头状瘤切除术

hepatectomy

肝切除术

segmental hepatectomy

肝段切除术

hepatobiliary exploration

肝胆管探查术

hepaticotomy

肝管切开术

cholecystectomy

胆囊切除术

laparoscopic cholecystectomy

腹腔镜胆囊切除术

cholangiography

胆道造影术

cholecystostomy

胆囊造口术

choledochostomy

胆总管造口术

cholecystoenterostomy

胆囊空肠吻合术

biliary enterostomy

胆肠内引流术

intrahepatic biliary duct drainage

肝胆管引流术

portal systemic venous shunt disconnection

门体静脉断流手术

choledoch end-to-end anastomosis

胆总管对端吻合术

choledochol cyst excision

胆总管囊肿切除术

transcystic duct cholangiography

经胆囊管胆道造影

portal vena cava anastomosis

门腔静脉吻合术

portosystemic stentsgunts

门体静脉分流术

total pancreaticoduodenectomy

全胰十二指肠切除术

pancreatectomy

胰切除术

splenectomy

脾切除术

gastrectomy

胃切除术

partial gastrectomy

胃部分切除术

cystogastrostomy

胃空肠吻合术

proximal gastrectomy and esophagogastrostomy

近端胃切除和食管胃吻合术

subtotal gastrectomy and gastrojejunostomy

胃大部切除和胃空肠吻合术

subtotal gastrectomy and gastroduodenostomy

胃大部切除和胃十二指肠吻合术

total gastrectomy esophagojejunostomy

全胃切除食管空肠吻合术

Roux-en-Y choledochojejunostomy

Roux-en-Y 胆总管空肠吻合术

pyloroplasty

幽门成形术

partial colectomy

结肠部分切除术

right colectomy

右半结肠切除术

transverse colectomy

横结肠切除术

enterostomy

肠造口术

permanent ileostomy

永久性回肠造口

double barrel transverse colostomy

横结肠双腔造口术

injured colon exteriorization

结肠损伤处外置造口术

circumferential hemorrhoidectomy

内痔环型切除术

appendicectomy

阑尾切除术

herniorrhaphy

疝修补术

indirect inguinal hernia hernioplasty

腹股沟斜疝修补术

direct inguinal hernia hernioplasty

腹股沟直疝修补术

perianal abscess incision and drainage

肛周脓肿切开引流术

anus and rectum(Mile's operation) abdominoperineal resection

经腹会阴直肠肛管切除术

seton therapy

挂线疗法

hemorrhoidectomy

痔切除术

fissure excision

肛裂切除术

drainage of the abscess

脓肿引流

subphrenic abscess drainage

膈下脓肿引流术

paraaortic lymphadenectomy

腹主动脉旁淋巴结清扫术

retroperitoneal tumors resection

腹膜后肿瘤切除术

exploratory laparotomy

开腹探查术

ligation of lower oesophageal veins

低位食管静脉结扎

high ligation of great saphenous vein and excision of varicosa veins

大隐静脉高位结扎及曲张静脉切除术

7. urinary surgery
泌尿外科

nephrectomy

肾切除术

cystoplasty

膀胱成形术

cystostomy

膀胱造口术

nephrostomy

肾造口术

nephrolithotomy

肾石切除术

orchiectomy

睾丸切除术

prostatectomy

前列腺切除术

renal biopsy

肾活检

renal transplantation

肾移植

urethra-lithotomy

输尿管结石切除

urethroplasty

尿道成形术

vasoligation

输精管结扎术

transurethral resection of bladder tumor(TURBT)

经尿道膀胱肿瘤切除

8. orthopaedics
骨科

knee joint fusion

膝关节融合术

osteochondroma excision

骨软骨瘤切除术

thigh amputation

大腿截肢术

leg amputation

小腿截肢术

forearm amputation

前臂截肢术

knee meniscectomy

膝关节半月板切除术

external fixation

外固定

internal fixation

内固定

knee arthroscope operation

膝关节镜手术

popliteal cyst resection

腘窝囊肿切除术

arthrodesis

关节固定术

curettage if bone tumor

骨瘤刮除术

fasciotomy

筋膜切开术

excision of bone tumor

骨瘤切除术

free skin graft

自由皮瓣移植

plaster splintage

石膏夹板固定

plaster cast

石膏管形

reduction of the fracture

骨折复位

repair if ligament

韧带修补

reduction of joint dislocation

关节脱位复位

replantation if digit

断指再植

skeletal traction

骨牵引

tenorrhaphy

腱缝合术

hallux valgus orthomorphia

拇外翻矫形

leg elongation

小腿延长术

achilles tendon lengthening

跟腱延长术

joint open drainage

关节切开引流术

severed limbs replantation

断肢再植术

spinal canal anterolateral decompression

椎管侧前方减压术

posterior instrumentation and fusion for idiopathic scoliosis

脊柱侧弯矫形术

lumbar spine decompression and fusion

腰椎减压融合术

nucleus pulposus of lumbar intervertebral disk resection

腰椎间盘髓核摘除术

excision of chondroma

软骨瘤刮除术

proximal humerus tumor excision

肱骨近端肿瘤切除术

metacarpophalangeal joint arthroplasty

掌指关节成形术

femoral neck fracture hollow needle internal fixation

股骨颈骨折空心钉内固定术

femoral tuberositas fracture internal fixation

股骨粗隆骨折切开内固定术

king-steelquis semipelvectomy

半骨盆切除术

clavicle fracture open reduction and internal fixation

锁骨骨折切开复位内固定术

Galeazzi's fracture open reduction and internal fixation

盖氏骨折切开复位内固定术

scaphoid fracture open reduction and internal fixation

腕舟骨骨折切开复位内固定术

ruptured Achilles tendon repair

跟腱断裂修补术

prosthetic replacement for joint

人工关节置换术

dislocation of elbow joint open reduction

肘关节脱位切开复位术

dislocation of hip joint open reduction

髋关节脱位切开复位术

patellar fracture open reduction and internal fixation

髌骨骨折切开复位内固定术

femoral head prosthetic replacement

人工股骨头置换术

hip join prosthetic replacement

人工全髋关节置换术

intertrochanteric fracture of femurγ-pinl fixation

股骨粗隆骨折 γ 钉内固定术

knee posterior synosteotomy

膝后关节囊切开术

tibial(fibula) fracture open reduction and internal fixation

胫(腓)骨骨折切开复位内固定术

tibial condyle fracture open reduction and internal fixation

胫骨髁骨骨折切开复位内固定术

cervical vertebral canal posterior decompression and enlarging plastic operation

颈椎后路减压及椎管扩大成形术

open reduction and internal fixation of humerus fracture

肱骨骨折切开复位内固定术

femoral neck fracture close reduction and internal fixation by compressive screws

股骨颈骨折闭合复位加压螺纹钉内固定术

femoral shaft fractures internal fixation by interlocking intramedullary nail

股骨干骨折交锁髓内钉内固定术

tibial shaft fractures interlocking intramedullary nail fixation

胫骨干骨折交锁髓内钉内固定术

ulnar and radial shaft fracture open reduction and internal fixation

尺骨桡骨骨干骨折切开复位内固定术

Colles' fracture open reduction and internal fixation

桡骨远端骨折(Colles')切开复位内固定术

metacarpal bone fracture open reduction and internal fixation

掌骨骨折切开复位内固定术

fracture of phalanx of finger open reduction and internal fixation

指骨骨折切开复位内固定术

surgery neck fracture of humerus open reduction and internal fixation

肱骨外科颈骨折切开复位内固定术

dislocation of the acromioclavicular joint open reduction and internal fixation

肩锁关节脱位切开复位内固定术

ulnar olecranal fracture open reduction and internal fixation

尺骨鹰嘴骨折切开复位内固定术

femoral shaft fracture open reduction and plate internal fixation

股骨干骨折切开复位接骨板内固定术

medial、lateral collateral（cruciate）ligament of knee joint repair

膝关节内、外侧副（交叉）韧带断裂修复术

9. gynaecology and obstetrics
妇产科

abdominoscopy

腹腔镜检查

abdominouterectomy

腹式子宫切除术

hysteroscopy

宫腔镜检查

myomectomy

子宫肌瘤挖除术

oophorectomy

卵巢切除术

oophorocystectomy

卵巢囊肿切除术

salpingostomy

输卵管复通术

subradical hysterectomy

次广泛子宫切除术

cesarean section

剖宫产术

vaginal hysterectomy

经阴道子宫切除术

amniocentesis

羊膜穿刺术

dilatation of the cervix

宫颈扩张术

cervicectomy

子宫颈切除术

excision of Bartholin cyst

巴氏腺囊肿切除术

culdocentesis

后穹隆穿刺术

induction of labor

引产术

hysterectomy

子宫切除术

ovarian cystectomy

卵巢囊肿切除术

salpingectomy

输卵管切除术

uterine curetlage

刮宫术

sterilization

绝育术

repair of laceration of cervix

子宫颈裂伤修补术

vulvectomy

外阴切除术

cervical polypectomy

宫颈息肉切除术

episiotomy

会阴切开术

adnexopexy

子宫附件固定术

tube ligation

输卵管结扎

colporrhaphia anterior-posterior

阴道前后壁修补术

ovary tumor rebulking operation

卵巢癌肿瘤细胞减灭术

total hysterosalpingo-oophorectomy

全子宫双附件切除术

subtotal hysterosalpingo-oophorectomy

次全子宫加双附件切除术

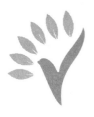

第二部分

手术室常用英文例句

一、Common communication sentences

（手术室）日常通用英文语句

1. common sentences of medical staff

（手术室）医务常用语句

What can I do for you?

有什么可以帮助您吗？

Can/May I help you?

我可以提供帮助吗？

(Is there) anything I can do for you?

您有什么需要我帮助的吗？

What's up? /What's wrong? / What happened?

您怎么啦？

What's your trouble/matter/problem?

您遇到什么麻烦啦？

Please wait a few minutes. /Wait here for a while.

请稍等一下。

Would you please wait a moment?

您可以稍等一下吗？

Follow me. / This way, please.

请往这边走。

Pardon? /Would you mind repeating it again?

再说一遍好吗？

You got it? /Can you catch me? / Do you understand me?

您明白我的意思吗？

It's not that serious. /It's curable/treatable.

没那么严重。/（这个疾病）可以治得好。

You can get a quick recovery.

您会很快好起来的。

Cheer up. /Keep smiling. / Don't lose heart.

别泄气，振作起来。

You are welcome.

不用谢（不客气）。

How long have you been ill? /How long have you been like this?

您病了多久了？

Be quiet. /Keep silent. /Please keep quiet.

请保持安静。

I will do/try my best.

我会尽最大努力。

Do you feel chest tightness?

您感到胸闷吗？

I will solve it.

我来解决。

Very good!

非常好！

You did very well.

您做得非常好。

Come on.

加油。

Listen! Look! Trust me!

听着！看着！相信我！

It's not like that.

并非像您说的那样。

I'll be back soon.

我很快回来。

Please hold on.

坚持住。

You have a beautiful baby.

您生了一个漂亮宝宝。

She looks healthy.

她看起来很健康。

How are you feeling now?

您现在感觉如何？

Tell me what the pain is like?

告诉我是一种怎样的痛？

Do you get this pain all the time?

您经常这样痛吗？

Wish you a good day.

祝您今天顺利。

That's all right.

没关系。

It's my pleasure.

这是我的荣幸。

Yes, I know. I am very sorry.

是的，我知道。我很抱歉。

OK，I have done/finished.

好了，完成啦。

Thank you for your understanding.

谢谢您的理解。

It's a piece of cake.

小意思。

Of course! /You bet! / No problem!

没问题，当然可以！

Good-bye.

再见。

Excuse me.

请原谅。

Good luck to you.

祝您好运。

Take good care of yourself.

请您多保重。

Cheer up，I think everything will be okay/fine.

振作起来吧，我想一切会好的。

I am so sorry to hear that you don't feel well.

听说您感到不舒服，我很难过。

Take it easy.

别着急，放心好了。

Don't worry about it.

别为那件事操心。

Don't take it so much to your heart.

别把那件事放在心上。

It's just one of those things.

这是无可避免的事。

It can't be helped.

这是没办法的。

Let's hope for the better.

乐观些,想开些。

It's difficult to say exactly what's wrong just now.

现在还不好说是什么问题。

It doesn't sound serious.

看起来病情并不严重。

Please don't be afraid, it is a minor operation.

请不要担心,只是一个小手术。

There is nothing to worry about.

没什么可担心的。

I am sure you'll be fine.

我确信您会好的。

I hope you'll be well soon.

希望您早日恢复健康。

It won't take long to recover.

很快就会恢复了。

2. common sentences of patients (手术室)病人常用语句

I feel nervous.

我感到紧张。

I'm not feeling well today.

今天我觉得很不舒服。

I have a cough.

我咳嗽。

I feel vertigo/dizzy/feverish/shivery/weak/sleepy/nausea/ itching/like vomiting.

我感到眩晕/晕头转向/发热/寒战/虚弱/瞌睡/恶心/痒/想吐。

I feel painful on motion.

我一动就疼。

I feel no pain.

一点也不疼。

I hate injection.

我讨厌打针。

I just got used to it.

我习惯了。

Has it been finished?

已经完成了吗？

Are you sure?

你确定吗？

How much will it take?

需要多少钱？

Thank you for your patience.

谢谢您耐心的工作。

I have no insurance. I pay for it myself.

我没有保险。我是自费的。

The doctor told me that I was cured.

医生说我已经痊愈了。

What shall/should I do?

我该怎么做?

I don't worry about it at all.

我一点也不担心。

I am so scared.

我非常害怕。

二、Preoperative interview
术前访视

1. greeting and contact
问候与接触

Hello, I am the nurse of operating room.

您好,我是手术室的护士。

Hello, my name is . . . , you can call me . . .

你好,我是……,您可以称呼我……。

What's your name? /Can I have your name?

请问您叫什么名字?

What's the matter with you?

您哪儿不舒服?

Can you tell me what's wrong with you, please?

请告诉我您怎么啦?

You don't look well. Is there anything wrong?

您看起来气色不好,哪里不舒服?

Do you feel weak?

您感觉虚弱吗?

Do you feel tired recently?

最近您感觉很疲劳吗?

How is your appetite? Any vomiting?

您的胃口怎样? 呕吐吗?

Do you have a good appetite?

您食欲好吗？

Did you sleep well?

您睡得好吗？

Did you have sleeplessness frequently?

您是否时常失眠？

Do you know that you are scheduled to have an operation tomorrow?

您知道自己明天要做手术吗？

You will have an operation tomorrow.

您明天被安排了手术。

I'm coming to acquire your basic condition and inform you some preparatory work, along with circumstance of the operating room.

我这次来是为了了解您的基本情况，并向您介绍手术室环境和术前准备。

2. history consulting
病史询问

How long have you felt sick?

您病了多久了？

What disease have you had before?

过去您患过什么疾病？

Have you had operation before?

您过去做过手术吗？

Have you ever had any surgery? What for?

您做过什么手术吗？是什么原因做手术呢？

Do you have diabetes, heart disease, or high blood pressure?

您有糖尿病、心脏病或高血压吗?

Have you had any serious accidents or diseases?

您有过严重的疾病史或受伤史吗?

Did you have any cardiac trouble?

以前有过心脏问题吗?

Have you ever had blood transfusion?

您曾经输过血吗?

Are there any medicines that you can't take?

您有哪些药不能吃吗?

Do you smoke? How much do you smoke per day?

您抽烟吗? 一天抽多少?

How long have you been smoking?

您抽烟有多久了?

Do you drink alcohol? How often do you drink?

您喝酒吗? 多久喝一次?

How much do you weigh? Has your weight changed recently?

您的体重是多少? 最近有变化吗?

Do you have any skin problems? Such as itching, sores, rashes or lumps?

您的皮肤最近有什么问题吗? 比如瘙痒、疮、皮疹或肿块?

Have you ever been unconscious for an injury?

您曾经有过外伤所致意识丧失吗?

Have you ever had headaches? What do you think causes them?

您头痛吗? 您认为是什么引起的呢?

Do you have any trouble with your noses or sinuses?

您的鼻子或鼻窦有什么问题吗?

Does your nose get stuffy or bleeding?

您是否有鼻塞或鼻出血方面的问题?

Do you have a history of sinus infections, nasal fracture or nasal injuries?

您有没有鼻窦感染、鼻骨骨折或鼻外伤的病史?

Have you been told that you snore?

有人告诉您您睡觉打鼾吗?

Does it hurt when you open your mouth?

您张嘴痛吗?

Do you have cavities or any other dental problems?

您有虫牙或其他牙齿问题吗?

Do you have any loose teeth?

您有松动的牙齿吗?

Do you wear dentures?

您戴假牙吗?

Do you have sore throat?

您咽喉痛吗?

Do you get hoarse? How long have you had hoarseness?

您声音嘶哑吗? 多久了?

Do you have difficulty in swallowing?

您是否有吞咽困难?

Do you choke when you eat solid food?

您吃硬质食物是否会噎住?

Do you wear glasses or contact lenses?

您戴框架或隐性眼镜吗?

What troubles do you have during the pregnancy?

这次怀孕有何不适?

Do you have any dizziness, nausea, vomiting, headaches or blurring of vision?

您有头晕、恶心、呕吐、头痛或视力模糊的现象吗?

What's wrong with your baby?

您的小宝宝有什么问题吗?

Does he eat any other food besides milk?

他除了吃奶以外还吃其他的吗?

Does your child get a cold?

您的孩子感冒了吗?

How much has he been coughing?

他咳得厉害吗?

Does he have any sputum?

他有痰吗?

Does your child ever become pale suddenly?

您的孩子是否有过突然脸色发白的情况?

Is the child anaemic?

孩子贫血吗?

What's troubling your eyes?

您的眼睛有什么不舒服吗?

Is it a shooting pain or burning pain?

是刺痛还是灼痛?

Do you have double vision or blurry vision?

您是否有复视或视物模糊?

Was there any drainage from your eyes?

您的眼睛有分泌物吗?

Dose light bother your eyes?

您的眼睛畏光吗?

Are you near-sighted or far-sighted?

您有近视或远视吗?

How is your hearing?

您的听力如何?

Do you have trouble in breathing?

您的呼吸有问题吗?

When and how did you notice a lump in your breast?

您什么时候以及如何发现自己乳腺有肿块的?

Have you ever noticed any tenderness or lump in your underarm area?

您曾注意到自己腋下有压痛或肿块吗?

Has anyone in your family had breast cancer?

您有乳腺癌的家族史吗?

Do you have abdominal pain? Which position?

您腹痛吗? 在哪个位置?

Whenever you feel pain, you can do deep breathing to relax.

感觉痛的时候您可以通过深呼吸来帮助您放松。

You could also bend your knees so that you can feel less painful.

您也可以弯曲膝盖,这样可以感到疼痛减轻一些。

The doctor cannot give you any painkiller because it might hide your symptoms.

医生现在还不能给您止痛药,因为它会掩盖您的症状。

The doctor has prescribed medication for your abdominal pain. The nurse will give you an injection later.

医生已经为您开了止痛药,护士等会就来为您注射。

If you think you need one, please ask the doctor and he can prescribe a premed injection before you come to the operating room.

您如果需要可以让医生在术前给您开镇静药。

Do you have any secretions from the ears?

您的耳朵有分泌物吗?

Does the earache occur deep inside or just the orifice of your ear?

耳痛是发生在耳朵深处还是在耳朵口呢?

Can you tell me what your question is?

您能告诉我您想要问的问题吗?

Is there anything else that you don't understand?

还有哪些您不清楚的?

If you have any problems, please don't be hesitating to tell me or anyone of us.

如果您还有什么问题,请不要犹豫,您可以问我或其他护士。

If we can't help you, we will find someone who can.

即使我们无法解决,我们也会找其他人来帮您解决问题。

3. health education of operation
手术健康教育

I come here to visit you and let you know some attentions about surgery.

我过来看望您,并告知您关于手术的一些注意事项。

We are going to do the operation tomorrow. I hope you won't be nervous.

明天我们就要安排您做手术了,希望您不要紧张。

You are going to have general anesthesia, so you won't feel pain during the operation.

您将进行的是全麻,所以手术期间您不会觉得痛。

Have you signed your consent yet? If not, the surgeon will talk with you about the surgery.

您在手术同意书上签字了吗? 如果还没有,将会有医生找您谈话的。

A surgeon will come to see you before surgery and explain what he is going to do and ask you to sign a consent form.

外科医生将在手术之前过来看您并向您解释他将做的事情,同时会要求您签手术同意书。

You are scheduled for the first operation which will start at eight o'clock tomorrow.

您的手术安排在明天第一台,早上八点钟开始。

You have be scheduled the second/third surgery.

您被安排在第二台/三台手术。

It's a long wait and you might be hungry and thirsty. If you feel uncomfortable, please tell your primary nurse.

长时间等待,您可能会感到饥饿和口渴。如果不舒服,请及时告知您的责任护士。

You can't eat or drink anything since you feel very hungry and thirsty.

即使您觉得很饿或口渴,仍然不能吃喝任何东西。

If you feel thirsty, you can just moisten your lips with cotton swab.

如果您觉得口渴难耐,您可以用棉签湿润口唇。

Our staff will pick you up around ×× o'clock to the operating room. Please stay here to wait for us.

我们的员工会在 ×× 点左右接您到手术室,在此之前请不要离开。

The anesthesiologist will come to see you and ask you some questions right away.

麻醉师待会会来看您并询问您一些问题。

As you're going to have a general anesthesia, you won't have any feel.

由于您施行的是全身麻醉,您不会有任何感觉。

Take it easy, Mr. Zhao. The surgeon who is going to give you the operation is very experienced and considerate. Everything will work out fine.

别紧张,赵先生。为您做手术的医生经验很丰富,且考虑周全。一切都会顺利进行的。

As you're going to have a local anesthesia, you could communicate with us during the operation.

由于您施行的是局部麻醉,在术中您是可以与我们沟通的。

You cannot eat or drink anything after ×× pm last night.

您需要在手术前一天晚上××点钟后禁食禁水。

Please put on the hospital dress and remove your false teeth, glasses and jewelry before operation.

手术前请换上病服,摘掉您的假牙、眼镜和首饰。

Don't take valuables into operation room.

不要将贵重物品带进手术室。

Please take X ray and CT to operation room for doctor's reference during the operation.

请将您的 X 片和 CT 片带到手术室,以供医生在手术过程中作为参考。

The doctor who will operate on you is very experienced and considerate.

给您做手术的医生是富有经验和细致耐心的。

If you have any discomfort in the operating room, please tell us in time and we can help you.

如果您感到任何不舒适,请及时告知我们,我们将帮助您。

The operation starts at nine o'clock in the morning, but our support staff will pick you up to the operation waiting room at eight o'clock.

手术上午九点开始,但我们的员工将在八点过来接您到术前等待间。

In the preoperative waiting room, nurses will look after you and you can tell them if you feel any discomfort.

在术前等待间,护士会照顾您,如果您有任何不适,请告知她们。

We'll prepare a warm and comfortable bed for you in the operating room.

我们会为您准备一张温暖舒适的手术床。

You will go to the operating room on a trolley.

我们会用平车将您护送到手术室。

Your primary nurse will give you an enema tonight.

今晚您的责任护士将给您灌肠。

Try to hold it in for a few minutes before you expel it.

您要先憋几分钟后再排便。

If you feel a distention or other discomfort, please tell the nurse in time.

如果在操作中,您有肚子胀或任何不适,请立即告知护士。

Your primary nurse will put a tube into your bladder through urethral to help you pass the urine and protect your bladder during the operation.

您的责任护士将会给您进行导尿——将一根导管经过尿道插入膀胱,帮助您排尿,同时在术中保护膀胱。

It may be uncomfortable, please be patient and you will get used to it after a while.

导尿会不舒服,但请您忍耐,过会儿就适应了。

You will have the results of your tests later today, and the doctor will come and tell you.

化验结果将在今天晚点出来,医生会过来告诉您。

A nurse will come and prepare you for the operation on time.

护士会按时为您准备手术的一切物品。

The nurse will conduct an enema for you at 8:00 pm.

护士在晚上 8:00 为您进行灌肠。

You'll have a urinary catheter to help you pass the urine during the operation.

您需要留置导尿管来帮助您在术中排尿。

It is a little tough somehow, but you must learn to be accustomed to it for the security of the surgery.

这的确会有点难受,但为了手术安全您必须要学会适应它。

You can start to have some liquid diet after you pass the gas.

等您开始排气以后就能进食流质食物了。

After surgery you can only have fluid for a couple of days and you will have intravenous fluid.

手术后前几天您只能进食流质饮食并要进行静脉输液。

You should try to turn over slightly which will promote your bowel movement and eliminate the gas in the abdomen.

术后几天您可以轻轻翻身,以促进肠蠕动、减少肠胀气。

You should start to use a bedpan now in order to accustom yourself to it.

您现在就应练习床上使用便盆来帮助术后尽快适应。

As you'll be a little bit weak after the surgery, it's difficult for you to get up to go to the toilet.

因为您术后会比较虚弱,起身如厕会有些困难。

After the operation, an anesthetist will come back with you and observe you on the way.

手术结束后,麻醉医生会和您一起回来并一路观察。

The doctor will come to see you and explain your conditions during the operation.

医生在术后会来看您并向您解释术中的情况。

Then try to have a good sleep and wish you a successful operation!

那么祝您一夜安睡,手术顺利!

It's hard to tell you how long you will stay in the operating room. It will depend on operating procedure and your recovery from anesthesia.

很难告诉您手术要多久。这取决于手术的进程以及您从麻醉中苏醒的时间。

You will probably return to this room in the afternoon.

您可能要在下午回到病房。

After the surgery you will spend a few hours in the recovery room.

手术结束后您要在恢复室休息几个小时。

After your condition is stable, you will come back here, probably after ✕✕ pm.

等您情况稳定后就会回到这里，大概是下午✕✕点钟以后了。

When you come back, you will still be very sleepy.

等您回来的时候您还在嗜睡状态。

Abdominal surgery may be painful, be sure to tell the nurse if you have pain and she will give you some painkillers for it.

腹部手术会有些痛，当您痛的时候就告诉护士，她会给您止痛药的。

You need to learn to cough, breath deeply and do leg exercises to prevent postoperative complications.

您需要学会咳嗽、深呼吸和腿部练习来预防术后并发症。

The complications include some problems with lungs and legs circulation due to anesthesia and bed rest.

这些并发症包括由麻醉和长期卧床引起的肺部和腿部血流不畅的问题。

As soon as you awake, we will be saying "take a deep breath, cough", in order to prevent pneumonia.

当您醒来时，我们指导您"咳嗽、深呼吸"来预防肺炎。

The nurse will help you get out of bed the next day to promote blood circulation of your lower body.

第二天护士还会帮您下床活动，以促进下肢血液循环。

三、Nursing in waiting room
等待间护理

Glad to meet you.

认识您很高兴。

I am the primary nurse of the preoperative waiting room.

我是等待间的责任护士。

I will be accompanied with you before the operation and you could ask me anything about the surgery.

在手术前我将会一直陪伴您,关于手术任何问题您都可以问我。

Please put on this operating cap.

请戴上这顶手术帽。

What is your name please?

请问您叫什么?

Let me check your wrist band.

让我核查一下您的手腕带。

Do you know what operation you will have?

您知道你将要做什么手术吗?

Did you sleep well last night?

您昨晚睡得好吗?

How is your sleep?

您睡眠怎样?

Did you drink any water?

您喝过水吗?

Have you eaten anything since last night?

从昨晚开始您吃过东西吗?

Do you feel cold?

您觉得冷吗?

What's wrong with you? /What is the problem with you?

您哪里不舒服?

Do you know the name of your operation?

您知道自己要做什么手术吗?

Do you know which part would be operated on?

您知道自己的手术部位吗?

Is there any operation mark on your body?

您身上有手术部位标记吗?

Does your doctor mark on your operative part?

您的管床医生在您手术部位做标记了吗?

You looks worried. Do you have any concerns?

您看起来有点焦虑,您有什么顾虑吗?

Mr. Li, I am going to take your vital signs.

李先生,我要为您测量生命体征。

The vital signs include temperature, heart rate, respiration rate and blood pressure.

生命体征包括体温、心率、呼吸频率和血压。

Now, please put the thermometer under your arm.

请将体温计夹在您的腋下。

Your temperature is normal.

您的体温是正常的。

Put your arm out, I'll check your pulse rate.

请伸出手臂,我给您测量脉搏。

I have checked your respiration without telling you so that breathing would be more nature.

我测呼吸时没告诉您,这样您呼吸会更自然。

I will roll up your sleeves to check your blood pressure.

我要将您的袖子挽上去以便为您测量血压。

Your blood pressure is one hundred and eighty over one hundred and ten mmHg. That's moderately high.

您的血压是 180/110 mmHg,有点高。

Did you take pills this morning?

您早上服药了吗?

You look pale. Are you in pain or uncomfortable?

您脸色苍白,您觉得哪里痛或不舒服吗?

You should lie in bed quietly, and try to relax and don't be too nervous.

您应该静卧、放松,不要太紧张。

Have you vomited?

您呕吐了吗?

Tilt your head aside and breath deeply in case of choking.

请将您的头偏向一边,深呼吸以免呛咳窒息。

Let me measure your blood glucose.

我要为您测量一下血糖。

Right now your blood glucose is 3.4 mmol/L, too low to maintain your body functioning basically.

您的血糖现在只有 3.4 mmol/L,太低了以至于不能维持您身体的基本机能。

I will give you the preoperative IV treatment to provide you energy.

术前我将给您静脉输液来为您提供能量。

The doctor has prescribed the IV treatment with glucose in it to alleviate your conditions of low blood glucose.

医生已经开具医嘱，给您输入葡萄糖来缓解您的低血糖症状。

Have you felt any amniotic fluid escaping?

您破水了没有？

Do you feel uterine contraction?

您感到宫缩了吗？

How long is the interval between contractions now?

现在收缩的间隙时间有多长？

What else do you feel?

你还感到些什么？

How long have you had the chest pain?

您胸痛有多久了？

Is the pain radiating to your shoulder?

疼痛辐射到您的肩部吗？

Do you feel weak and dizzy?

您感到虚弱和头晕吗？

Do you have a fever and headache?

您感到发烧和头疼吗？

Do you feel dehydrated?

您有脱水的感觉吗？

I need to examine you.

让我检查一下。

Try to keep relax and keep calm.

尽量放松，保持镇静。

There is nothing to worry about.

没什么可担心的。

Don't worry. You couldn't help it.

别着急,你自己也没有办法。

It's hard to tell what the problem is right now.

现在还说不好到底是什么问题。

These tubes are very important to you, though they make you uncomfortable.

尽管这些导管让您感到有点不舒服,但它们对您很重要。

The urinary tube makes you feel strange somehow, you will feel as you want to pass urine.

尿管多少会让您有点不舒服,您会觉得有点尿意。

Please do not worry about the passing urine which has been collected in the bag attached with the tube.

请不要担心排尿问题,所有的尿液都会收集到集尿袋里。

Do you want me to give you another blanket to keep warm?

您需要我给您加一条毛毯保暖吗?

Do you want to raise the pillow higher?

您的枕头需要抬高吗?

Do you need me to adjust the operating bed to make you feel better?

您需要我调节手术床让您感觉好受一点吗?

Maybe you have laid on your back too long which makes you feel uneasy.

也许是因为您平躺太久了才感觉不舒服。

Would you want me to help you to change your position?

我帮您换个体位,好吗?

Do you feel better now?

您感觉好些了吗?

You will be sent to the operating room when it is prepared well.

手术间准备好以后就会送您进去。

The families are not allowed to enter into the operating area.

家属不能进入手术区域。

Patients need to stay in the observation room until they are fully awake.

患者在完全清醒前需要在观察室留观。

There are special staff who will take good care of him and send him back to the ward.

那里会有专职人员悉心照顾他并送他回病房。

Please wait in the waiting area for the convenience of intraoperative conversation.

请在家属等待区等候，方便术中谈话。

The doctor may communicate with you about the concerned information of the patient during the operation.

医生在手术中可能需要与您沟通一些与手术患者相关的问题。

The removed tissues would be sent to the pathology room directly.

切除的组织会直接送到病理室。

The surgeon will show you the diseased tissue and talk with you about the further therapeutic regimen of the patient.

外科医生会给您看病变组织并和您谈论患者进一步的治疗方案。

It should take a few days to get the normal pathology result.

常规病理结果要等几天才能出来。

The surgeon will inform you when the operation is finished.

手术结束后医生会通知您。

The procedure has much less risk when compared with the surgery because the incision is relatively minimal.

这种手术伤口很小，比外科手术风险小多了。

I'm sure you'll recover quickly.

我相信您一定很快会恢复。

The operating team consists of experienced experts.

手术团队都是有经验的专家。

Please trust our medical staff.

请相信我们医护人员。

Please lie down and watch TV for a moment, the nurse will push you to the operating room after they finish the work shift.

请躺下休息看一会电视,手术护士交完班后就会来推您去手术间。

Now I'm taking you into the operating room.

现在我推您进手术间。

As there are some emergency cases, you might be waiting for a longer time.

因为一些紧急情况的发生,您需要多等一会儿。

Wait a moment, please.

请等一等。

I will come right now.

我马上就来。

Sorry, you can't drink water, but I can moisten your lips to quench your thirst.

抱歉,您不能喝水,但我可以湿润您的嘴唇来缓解口渴。

I am sorry to hear that.

我很遗憾听到这个消息。

I am afraid you misunderstood.

恐怕您误会了。

I think you should talk with your attending doctor and make it clear.

我认为您应该与您的主治医生谈谈，把这弄清楚。

I understand what you are saying.

我确实理解您所说的一切。

I understand how is your feeling.

我完全理解您的感受。

I am sorry that you have to wait so long.

真对不起让您等这么长的时间。

I'm sorry to inform you that your surgery has to be canceled for some reasons.

很抱歉通知您，由于某些原因您的手术不得不取消。

The surgeon will explain it to you later.

医生一会儿会跟您解释。

I believe all these are concerning about your security.

我相信一切都是为了您的安全考虑。

I appreciate your supporting and understanding.

我很感激您的理解支持。

Please wait patiently.

请耐心等待一下。

Don't be afraid. I think you can stand it.

别害怕，我想您能承受得住。

Fate often makes fun of people. The most important thing for you now is to live bravely.

命运常常捉弄人，现在对您来说最重要的就是勇敢地活下去。

The most important thing is to adjust yourself and build up self-confidence.

最重要的事情是调整心态，树立信心。

How long have you had abdominal pain?

您腹痛有多长时间了？

Where does it hurt?

您哪里疼？

How were you injured?

您是怎么受伤的？

Did you lose a lot of blood?

您出血多吗？

Do you have fresh wounds or any breakage in your skin?

您身上有新伤口或皮肤破溃的地方吗？

When did it happen?

是什么时候发生的？

The wound is rather large, so the doctor will stitch it up.

这个伤口比较大，所以需要缝合。

It won't be painful. We will give you local anesthesia.

不会痛的，我们会给您做局部麻醉。

You should give all your valuable things to your families or friends for safe keeping.

为安全起见，您需要把您所有的贵重物品交给您家人或者朋友。

You are a brave boy/girl/man/woman.

您真是勇敢的人。

Don't worry.

不要担心。

There is no danger.

没有任何危险。

Relax and take a deep breath.

深呼吸，放轻松。

He encountered a traffic accident and has lost consciousness for about an hour.

他遇到车祸,昏迷了差不多一个小时。

The patient has massive hemorrhage, and we need surgery in no time.

这个病人大出血,我们需要立即将他送进手术室进行手术。

What is your baby's weight?

您的宝宝多重了?

How tall is your baby?

您的宝宝多高了?

Does he cough?

他有没有咳嗽?

Does he have a fever?

他有没有发烧?

Have you feed your baby the latest four hours?

最近四小时您有喂宝宝喝奶吗?

Don't cry, little baby, you are so cute and so brave.

不要哭,小宝贝,你真可爱、真勇敢。

It's the great love of parents all over the world.

可怜天下父母心。

The treatment of disease is a long period which need your cooperation.

疾病治疗是个长期过程,需要您长期配合。

You should be stronger to build a positive example for your kid.

为了给孩子树立一个好榜样,您更要坚强。

Your emotion will definitely influence the kid.

您的情绪必定会影响到孩子。

The disease is inevitable for the growth of every kid.

每个孩子成长都免不了疾病的烦恼。

Are your families outside? We need her/him to sign the anesthesia consent.

您家人在外面吗? 我们需要找她/他签麻醉同意书。

OK, we would take him in, and please stay at the family waiting area.

好了,我们将带他进去,您可以在家属等待区等候。

四、Preoperative preparation for operating room

手术室术前准备

1. preparation and communication in operating room

入室准备与沟通

Sit up carefully, support yourself with your hands.

小心地坐起来,用手扶好了。

Move onto the operating bed slowly, and buttress with the fringe of the bed.

慢慢移到手术台上,扶着手术台边。

Take off your coat, cover it on your body, and then lie down carefully.

脱掉您的衣服,盖好被子,然后慢慢躺下来。

Please take off your clothes/trousers/shoes.

请脱下衣服/裤子/鞋子。

I'll keep you warm.

我会为您保暖的。

Please take off the shoes and lie down on your back.

请脱鞋上床,仰卧。

Do you feel cold? Now I'm covering you with the mattress which will keep you warm.

您觉得冷吗? 我现在拿被子给您盖上保暖。

Please unbutton your shirt.

请解开衣扣。

I have to tie up your left/right arm/legs in order to ensure your safety.

我必须对您的左/右胳膊/大腿进行约束，以保证您的安全。

It may be uncomfortable, but I have to.

可能会有些不舒服，但我必须这样做。

Too tight? All right, I'll loosen it.

太紧了？好的，我松开点。

You are going to have general anesthesia, so during the operation you will have no feeling.

您会全身麻醉，在手术期间不会有感觉。

Take it easy. The doctor who will operate on you is very experienced and considerate.

别担心，给您做手术的大夫很有经验和耐心。

It's hard to say. It depends on operation procedures and your recovery from the anesthesia. I imagine that it will take about × × hours.

这很难说。要看手术进展和您从麻醉中苏醒的情况，预计××个小时。

I will paste an electrode pad on your leg.

我将在您的腿上贴一个电极板。

It may be cold, and please be patient for a while.

可能会有点冰，请稍微忍耐一下，很快就好了。

I am going to put an electric tourniquet around your leg/arm, it will be tight.

我将在您的腿上或手臂上绑一个止血带，可能会有点紧。

Don't be nervous.

不要紧张。

Try to relax and keep calm.

尽量放轻松，保持镇静。

Thank you for your cooperation.

谢谢您的合作。

2. intravenous catheter and medication
静脉留置针与用药

I'll give you intravenous infusion.

我将要给您静脉输液。

There would be some pain when puncture, please cooperate with me, OK?

打针时有点痛，请您配合一下，可以吗？

Don't be afraid. It feels just like a mosquito bite. You're a brave boy/girl.

不要害怕，打针就像被蚊子咬一口，你是一个勇敢的男孩/女孩。

Spread out your hand, please.

请把手伸开。

In order to give you intravenous infusion during your operation, now I'm giving you a venipuncture and leave a detaining needle in your vein.

为了术中静脉输液，现在我要给您做静脉穿刺，还要留一个套管针在血管里。

I will insert a detaining needle into your vein in the wrist/elbow/foot/hand.

我需要插一个套管针到您的血管中,在您的手腕/手肘/脚/手。

I am going to put a tourniquet around your arm.

我接下来要绑一个止血带在你的手臂处。

You will feel tight and a small prick, please try and keep still for me.

你会感觉有点紧和有点疼,请尽量保持不动。

Please don't move.

请不要动。

I will try to do it carefully.

我会小心做的。

Please clench your fist.

请您握拳。

The cannula needle is a little thick and can be a bit painful.

套管针的针头有些粗,会有些疼。

I'm just going to disinfect your skin.

接下来我将给您皮肤进行消毒。

I am so sorry, I did a failed venipuncture, and it's a pity to tell that you have to get another one.

非常抱歉,我穿刺失败,您不得不再进行一次穿刺。

You can loose your fist now.

您现在可以松开拳头了。

It's OK. Now just lie down here and wait for the doctors.

好了,现在就好好躺着等手术医生过来。

This detaining needle can be detained for three days, so when you're back to your ward, you don't have to get venipuncture every day.

套管针三天有效,所以您回到病房后不需要每天都进行静脉穿刺了。

The fluids will provide energy for you.

输入的液体能为您提供能量。

The fluids can prevent electrolytic imbalances after operation.

输入的液体能预防术后电解质失衡。

Do you have any drug allergies?

您对什么药物过敏吗?

Are you allergic to any other medicine?

您对其他药物过敏吗?

When did you have the skin test?

您什么时候做的皮试?

Doctor Li, I need to check the result of skin test in electronic medical records.

李医生,我需要查看电子病历里面的皮试结果。

You need to confirm the skin test results of this patient with the ward nurse.

您需要与病房护士确认一下这个病人的皮试结果。

The result of the skin test is positive/negative.

皮试结果为阳性/阴性。

3. anesthesia
麻醉

I need to give you an arterial puncture.

我需要给您进行动脉穿刺。

If you have any questions about anesthesia, you can ask your anesthetist.

如果您对麻醉有什么问题，都可以问您的麻醉师。

If you feel uncomfortable, just tell me.

如果您觉得不舒服，就跟我说。

If you feel hurt, just tell me.

如果您觉得疼了，就跟我说。

Please lie on your left side (right side, back).

请左侧卧（右侧卧，平卧）。

Please bend your knees.

请屈膝。

Please relax the muscles of your legs.

请放松腿部肌肉。

Please lift your leg up slightly.

请稍稍抬起您的腿。

Please turn around and show me your back.

请转过来让我看看您的背。

Turn over and lie sideways. Keep stable or it may be dangerous.

翻身，侧躺着。保持不动，否则可能会有危险。

The doctor will do a lumbar/epidural anesthesia for you.

医生将给您打腰麻/硬膜外麻醉。

Please turn onto your left side for me.

请朝左侧躺着。

Please bend your knees as far as you can.

请您将膝盖尽量弯曲。

Please bend your head to touch your chest as far as you can.

请尽量低头触碰你的胸部。

I need your back curved as much as possible.

我需要您背部尽量弯曲。

I will put a pillow under your head, so it is more comfortable.

我会在你的头下面垫下枕头,这样会舒服很多。

You will feel pushing and a little pressure on your back.

您会感到背部有压力。

If you feel any uncomfortable, please never move and just tell us at once.

如果您感到任何不适,请千万不要动,只需立即告知我。

The doctor is going to disinfect your skin with iodine, it will be a little cold.

医生将用活力碘给您消毒,会感觉有些凉。

I'm ready for the injection.

我准备进针了。

The lumbar anaesthesia is finished.

腰麻已经完成了。

Please roll back onto your back.

请转过来平躺着。

You will need to stay in bed for 6 hours without pillow.

您需要去枕平卧 6 个小时。

If you want to sleep, please close your eyes and relax.

如果您想睡觉的话,那就请闭上眼睛放松。

Please lie down, anesthesia will start now.

请睡平,马上要开始进行麻醉了。

You won't feel any pain after the anesthesia.

麻醉后您就感觉不到疼。

Anesthesia can help you get through the operation safely.

麻醉能帮您安全顺利地度过手术。

I will give you an injection to numb the area.

我会给您注射一针,麻醉一下这个部位。

If 1 means no pain, and 10 means severe pain, what number would you give for your pain?

如果 1 代表不疼,10 代表剧烈疼痛的话,您对您目前的疼痛评多少分?

Let me take your blood pressure.

我给您量一下血压。

I am going to put a tourniquet around your upper arm.

我要在您的上臂绑一个血压计。

It will be very tight, but only for a moment.

会感觉很紧,但是一会儿就好了。

Please keep your arm still.

请保持你的手臂不动。

I am going to put these pads on your chest, they will be cold.

我将这些电极片贴在您的胸部,会感觉有点凉。

Please wear it and this is the oxygen saturation folder.

请戴上它,这是血氧饱和度测量夹。

Open your mouth and say "ah".

张开嘴说"啊"。

I'll look into your mouth.

我检查一下您的口腔。

4. preoperative catheterization、blood preparation
术前导尿、备血

I need to give you catheterization.

我要给你进行导尿。

I need to put a tube into your bladder to help you pass urine.

我要插一根管子到您的膀胱里帮助您排尿。

Don't be shy.

请不要害羞。

I've placed a sheet on your legs to protect your privacy.

我已放了一张床单在您的腿上来保护您的隐私。

You can't move until finish it.

在我完成前,您都不能动。

I will disinfect your vulva and it maybe cold.

我将给您的外阴消毒,可能会有点冷。

Please take a deep breath, and breathe out slowly through your mouth.

请深吸一口气,然后慢慢地用嘴呼出来。

You may feel the urge to urinate after applying the catheter, but you will get used to it soon.

您会感觉有尿意,不过很快就会适应的。

I need to remove your catheter.

我需要移除你的尿管。

I am going to draw a little blood from your arm.

我将要在您手臂上抽一点血。

We need some laboratory tests to help us make the diagnosis.

我们需要做几项化验来帮助诊断。

We need to get the blood type and a cross match for the preparation of blood transfusion.

我们需要得出您的血型以及交叉配血的结果，做好输血准备。

5. posture placement
体位安置

I will place the soft padding under your shoulder to prevent the injury of brachial plexus by potions.

我会在您肩下放置这个软垫，从而避免臂丛神经的损伤。

Stretch your forearms.

请伸展您的前臂。

Lift your left/right leg.

请抬起您的左/右腿。

The improved lithotomy position and the herringbone position were taken for laparoscopic radical resection of rectal carcinoma.

腔镜直肠癌手术采取改良截石位以及"人"字位的体位。

Proper position intervention is important for the prevention of postoperative complications.

正确的体位安置对预防术后并发症很重要。

I am going to place lithotomy position for you, please cooperate with me.

我将为您安置一个截石位，请您配合我。

Please open your legs slowly and keep relaxed.

请张开您的双腿，放轻松。

Put your legs on these two leg supports carefully.

请把双腿小心地放在这两个腿架上。

Don't be nervous and I would protect your privacy.

请不要紧张,我会保护好您的隐私。

Do you feel comfortable or is there any muscle pulling at your legs inside?

您觉得这样舒适吗? 或者您感到大腿内侧有肌肉拉扯感吗?

OK,I will replace it for you.

好,我将重新为您安置体位。

Please cooperate with me.

请配合我。

I need to set an easy prone position for you and you just need to hug a pillow under you.

我将为您安置一个简易的俯卧位,您只需要抱着身下的枕头。

You are placed a lateral potion/prone position for the operation.

为了手术的需要,您将被安置成侧卧位/俯卧位。

If you feel any uncomfortable during operation,don't move first and just tell me.

如果术中您有任何不舒适,首先请不要动,告知我就可以了。

As you feel stuffy,I will put the mask on your face to improve your breathing condition.

既然您觉得憋气,那么我给您戴上面罩来改善您的呼吸情况。

I am going to give you some oxygen,please put this oxygen mask over your face.

我接下来给您供氧,请将这个氧气罩戴上。

I have left you some space in case that you feel short of breath.

我给您留了点空间，免得您觉得喘不过气。

You could turn your head tightly if you feel your neck is stiff.

您如果觉得脖子僵硬，可以稍微转一下头。

Do you need a pillow to improve your comfort?

您需要垫个枕头来使自己感觉舒服点吗？

I'm going to place the thyroid position for you.

我需要为您安置甲状腺体位。

I will put a narrow pillow under your back and a cylindrical support under the neck.

我会在您背下垫上一个窄枕头，脖子下垫上一个柱状的支撑物。

Your neck will lean back which may feel uncomfortable.

您的脖子会向后仰，可能会感到不舒服。

The sandbags will hold your head in place.

沙袋会固定住您的头部。

The anaesthetist is preparing the medicine for you.

麻醉师正在为您准备药物。

The anaesthetist is injecting the medicine into you vessel which might make you feel a bit painful.

麻醉师将要给您用的静脉药会让您感觉到有点疼。

It won't last a long time before you fall asleep.

用不了多久您就会睡着的。

Please answer us when you hear our calling of your name.

醒来后听到我们叫您的名字请您应答。

We will also answer you some simple questions to judge your state of consciousness.

我们还会问您一些简单的问题来判断您的意识状态。

It is necessary that you do some required movement to tell us the recovering condition of your body.

还需要您配合做一些指令动作来让我们知晓您的身体恢复情况。

Now please be relax and listen to our command.

现在请放松听我们指令。

Please take a deep breath and breath out slowly through your mouth.

深吸气,再用嘴巴慢慢吐气。

Follow us to count numbers:ten,nine,eight,seven,six,five...

跟着我倒数,十、九、八、七、六、五……

Close your eyes and have a good sleep.

闭上眼睛好好睡一觉吧。

五、Intraoperative coordination
术中配合

1. common communication of operation
手术基本操作沟通

Could I scrub in?

我可以洗手上台了吗?

Let us do "Time Out" at first to ensure everything is all right.

让我们首先进行患者安全核查,来核对所有事项是否正确。

Do you have a spare operation room now?

请问现在可以安排手术房间吗?

It is local anesthesia, and please prepare some lidocaine for me.

手术的麻醉方式是局麻,请帮我备几支利多卡因。

Please connect the electrotome into this instrument.

请将电刀接到这个设备上。

Professor Li, let me help you to put on this sterile attire and gloves.

李教授,让我帮您穿上手术衣,戴上无菌手套吧。

What size of gloves do you need?

请问您戴什么号码的手套?

Do you need the scalpel?

您是需要手术刀吗?

What size of silk thread do you need?

您需要几号的丝线？

Please pass me blood vessel forceps.

请把血管钳递给我。

Doctor Li, please bound up the child's bleeding wound with gauze.

李医生，请把小孩出血的伤口用纱布包扎起来。

Do we need to give her urethral catheterization?

她需要导尿吗？

What size of catheter do you need? What about ××?

您需要几号尿管，××号行吗？

Please take care of electrocauterize, don't touch the skin around wound.

请小心使用电灼，注意不要碰到切口以外的皮肤。

Doctor performs operations with sterilized surgical instruments.

医生做手术需使用无菌手术器械。

Doctor Li, please keep your hands above your waist.

李医生，请把手保持在腰以上。

Don't turn your back on my sterile area, so as not to contaminate the sterile area.

不要将您的背对着无菌台，以防污染无菌区。

If you want to pass him with sterile attire, please back to back.

如果你们想递给他手术衣，请遵循无菌原则，后背对着后背交换。

If your attire is wet or contaminated, please change it.

如果您的手术衣湿了或者污染了，请更换。

Could you please let me go through? I need to move there.

麻烦请让一让,我要到那边去。

It may be necessary to have a blood transfusion during the operation.

手术中可能需要输血。

Please prepare ×× U whole blood and ×× mL plasma.

请准备×× U 的全血和××毫升的血浆。

We need prepare the auto-transfusion.

请准备自体血回输。

Doctor Li, let us check the blood.

李医生,我们来检查一下血。

Her temperature is low, and please keep the patient warm.

她的体温较低,给她供点暖。

Please give me a pack of hemostatic gauze.

请给我一包止血纱布。

Give me the cotton cushion, please.

请给我棉垫。

Gauze strip, please.

请给我纱条。

Wet cotton pads, gauze, forceps, please.

请给我湿棉垫、纱布、镊子。

Gauze with radiopaque line, please.

我需要显影纱布。

Please give me an injection syringe of 5/10/ 50 milliliter.

请给我一支 5 毫升/10 毫升/50 毫升的注射器。

This is suction machine to suck out excess blood and other fluids.

这是吸引器，用来吸引血和其他液体。

There is something wrong with the suction（apparatus），it stops working.

吸引（器）有点问题，没有吸力了。

Let me check it，it is empty/loose.

我来检查一下，它用完了/它接口松了。

OK，It is working.

好了，它开始工作了。

Please turn the power of electrotome up.

请把电刀功率调大点。

Turn it down.

调小点。

Please offer the bipolar coagulation forceps.

我需要双极电凝镊。

Which type do you want?

您需要哪种型号的？

Please aim the operational lamp at the field.

请把手术灯对准到术野中。

Put on a sterilized lamp holder.

请加一个无菌灯柄。

Scalpel，forceps，please.

请拿手术刀、镊子。

We should report to the head nurse first.

我们应该首先报告护士长。

Please don't make the dressing wet when you are disinfecting.

消毒时请不要将敷料打湿了。

Please add some muscle relaxant.

请加一点肌松药。

All the sterilized instruments are counted for four times during surgery to ensure that none have been left inside.

所有无菌器械在手术中要清点四遍,确保没有遗留任何东西。

This is the first counting.

这是第一次清点。

Let's do the last counting.

我们来做最后一次清点。

We should prepare rapid pathological examination of this tissue.

我们需要准备快速病理检查。

Put the specimen into the bag.

请将标本放置于标本袋中。

Please send the specimen with me together.

请和我一起去送检标本吧。

Let's check their information together.

我们一起来核对患者及其标本信息。

We need to change the way of surgery and talk with her/his families.

我们需改变手术方式,需要和她/他的家属谈谈。

It is bleeding, give me vascular suture.

正在出血,请给我血管缝合线。

How about 4-0 prolene?

4-0 血管线怎么样?

How about Vicryl suture?

薇乔线如何?

The light is weak, please replace it to light up the operative field.

灯光比较弱,请把灯移动到术野。

What is the gauge of this needle?

这个针是什么型号?

Safe first!

安全第一!

Please turn the power off.

请关掉电源。

Please help me to answer the phone.

请帮我接听电话。

I feel heavy dizzy and I am afraid I can't keep working.

我头很晕,恐怕我不能继续上台了。

All low-cost consumables are prepared?

所有低值耗材都准备好了吗?

We need a good exposure to surgical field.

我们需要充分暴露手术视野。

Vessel clamp, forceps, please.

请拿血管钳、镊子。

(Give me)stitch.

(给我)缝。

(Give him)scissors.

(给他)剪刀。

Knot tying with needle holder.

用持针器打结。

Ligation with ×× suture.

用××号线打结。

Ligation with double ×× suture.

用双××号线打结。

Keep suction.

一直吸。

Hold on please.

请坚持住。

Help me wipe my sweat.

帮我擦擦汗。

Help me wear my glasses.

帮我戴上眼镜。

Help me take off glasses.

帮我取下眼镜。

(Give me the)hemostatic materials.

(给我)止血材料。

Here you are.

给你。

Cut it into two pieces by scissors.

用剪刀剪成两半。

Doctor Li, please deliver this tissue to the specimen room.

李医生,请把标本送到标本间。

Have his head on his side, so that the saliva can run out without blocking his air passage.

让他的头侧着,使口水可以流出来,不致阻塞他的呼吸道。

(Place the patient in the)head-low position.

将病人置于头低位。

Elevate the foot of the bed.

抬高床腿。

Lower the operating bed please.

降低手术床。

Elevate the operational bed please.

升高手术床。

Adjust the bed to my opposite side.

将床向我对侧方向调整。

Clean the telescope.

擦拭镜头。

Two negative pressure absorbing balls.

两个负压引流球。

It's hard to give him intravenous infusion at this time, he had vasoconstriction due to the shock.

现在很难给他静脉输液,由于休克,他的血管收缩了。

We should assess his vital signs frequently.

我们需要经常观察他的生命体征。

We should maintain his urine output of at least 30 ml/hour.

我们要保证他的尿量每小时至少 30 毫升。

Be sure to keep the client warm, not too hot or too cold.

注意给病人保暖,不要太热太冷。

The blood pressure is low, and he needs blood transfusion right now.

血压有点低,他需要立即输血。

The child has been given infusion of 100 mL glucose solution.

这个患儿已输入 100 毫升的葡萄糖。

We should make everything clear when handing over to the next shift.

当我们和下一班护士交班时,所有东西都需要交接清楚。

There are 12 regular needles、8 special needles、10 pieces of large gauze、2 blades and 1 syringe on the operating table.

手术台上一共有 12 根普通针、8 根特殊针、10 块大纱布、2 个刀片和 1 套注射器。

The number of devices is correct and all the nuts are correct.

器械数量都是正确的,螺帽也都在。

The number of brain pads can't count clearly, so you can't take over now.

脑棉片的数量现在清点不清,因此你不能接班。

The patient is undergoing emergency treatment, so we can't take over the shift.

患者正在紧急抢救,我们暂时还不能交接班。

Let's check the name of the operation.

我们一起来核对一下手术名称。

2. intraoperative communication of various specialized surgeries
各专科手术的术中沟通

(1) ophthalmology
眼科

Now we begin to disinfect your skin, please close your eyes, please.

现在我们开始为您消毒皮肤了,请闭上眼睛。

We start to lay out sterile sheets around your eyes and keep still please.

我们开始在您的眼周铺置无菌布，请您保持不动。

Please lift your head a little and we will wrap your head with a sterile sheet.

请稍稍抬下头，我们将用无菌布包裹住您的头部。

Do you feel choked?

您感到憋气吗？

You are given a nasal oxygen tube with oxygen in it so you wouldn't feel choked.

给您使用了一根鼻氧管供给氧气，这样您就不会感到憋气了。

We have started the operation. If you have any discomfort during the operation, please speak directly. Don't move your body, especially your head.

我们已经开始手术了，如果术中您有任何不适，请直接说出来，不要随意动身体，尤其是您的头。

If you cough or sneeze, be sure to let us know in advance.

如果您要咳嗽或者打喷嚏，请一定提前告知。

The whole operation is performed under a microscope so that every step requires your full cooperation.

手术全程在显微镜下操作，所以任何一个步骤都需要您的全力配合。

Please open your eyes and I will place an eyelid opener for you.

请睁开眼睛，我要给您眼睛放置一个开睑器。

Now I am going to install the IOL and don't hold your breath.

现在我要安装人工晶体了，请不要憋气。

Please prepare more lidocaine.

请再准备一些利多卡因。

Has the cutting machine passed the test?

玻切机通过检测了吗？

Please prepare for the laser.

请准备激光机。

The patient has hemorrhage in the vitreous body cavity, and please prepare an electric coagulation wire.

患者玻璃体腔内有出血,请准备一个电凝线。

Please help her wear the laser protection glasses and get ready to start laser treatment.

请帮她戴上激光防护镜,现在开始激光治疗。

I need silicon oil and heavy water, please.

我需要硅油和重水。

It can increase the out flow of aqueous humor.

它能促进房水外流。

All the medicine should be divided clearly by the identifying during vitrorectomy.

玻切手术台上所有药品都需用标识区分清楚。

Please change the liquid storage box.

请更换储液盒。

The doctor is going to start the procedures now.

医生接下来要动手术了。

If you feel any pain, please tell me, and I will ask the doctor to give you some more local anesthetic.

如果您感到任何程度的疼,请告诉我,我会告诉医生给您进行更多的局部麻醉。

Just a few stitches left, and please hold on.

还有几针就缝完了,请再坚持一会。

The corneal suture has been removed completely.

角膜缝线已经给您彻底拆完了。

Please keep your eyes fixed on the upper right and I'll give you the injection right away.

请向右上方注视保持不动,我马上给您把药注射进去。

The medicine has been injected and don't splash water into eyes for next few days.

药已经注射进去了,接下来几天不能溅水到眼睛里。

The doctor has finished now and is putting a dressing on your eye.

医生已经完成了,现在正在给您眼睛贴敷料。

(2) otorhinolaryngology

耳鼻喉科

Please turn the head to the uninjured side and pay attention to protect it from compression.

请将患者头部偏向健侧,注意保护健侧耳朵以免受压。

Does the facial nerve monitor pass the test?

面神经监护仪通过检测了吗?

The patient's ossicular chain is intact.

患者的听骨链是完整的。

Does his ear have the cholesteatoma?

患者耳内有胆脂瘤吗?

Can you tell me how to connect the facial nerve monitor?

您可以告诉我怎么连接面神经监护仪吗?

The yellow line is inserted into orbicularisoris muscles, and another one is inserted into orbicularis oculi muscle.

这根黄色的线插入口轮匝肌,另一个则插入眼轮匝肌。

They are connected to the ground and negative poles.

他们分别连接在地线和负极。

Give me the probe pen to test the facial nerve.

给我探测笔检测一下面神经。

There is no response.

没有反应。

There is something wrong with the facial nerve monitor.

面神经监护仪出问题了。

I need a tiny needle electrome.

我需要微型针状电刀。

Is the nose power system ready?

鼻动力系统准备好了吗?

This drill bit can't work.

这个钻头磨不动了。

Drill bits need to be replaced regularly.

钻头需要定期更换。

Solid alex should be prepared in advance.

亚历克斯需要提前准备好。

Inject ×× drops of epinephrine into the saline solution.

滴××滴肾上腺素到生理盐水中。

When I'm grinding the bone, you have to use a syringe to pump water into the area to cool it down.

当我磨骨头的时候,您需要向磨的地方打水以此来降温。

You can pump the water a little slower.

您可以把打水的速度减慢一点。

Please prepare the otodynamic system.

请准备好耳动力系统。

A X-degree nasal endoscopy is required.

需要 X 度鼻内镜。

Two inflation sponges，please.

来两片膨胀海绵。

This child only need the adenoidectomy.

这名患儿只做腺样体切除术。

It needs the microlaryngoscope to see the epiglottis cyst.

需要显微喉镜才能看得见这个会厌囊肿。

Plasma ablation is more faster.

等离子消融得更快一些。

She had only bilateral tonsillectomy.

她只做双侧扁桃体切除术。

He needs to do the tracheotomy right now.

他现在需要立即进行气管切开术。

It is very dangerous for foreign bodies of trachea.

气管异物非常危险。

We put on this sterile microscopic set together.

我们一起来套这个显微镜无菌保护套。

Turn on the microscope light source.

打开显微镜光源。

The esophageal foreign body has been removed and given to his family.

食管异物已经取出来了，并交给了他的家属。

(3) stomatology
口腔科

Please turn your head to the left.

请把头转向左边。

Please keep your head straight.

请保持头直立。

Please tilt your head back.

请向后仰头。

Please tuck your chin.

请收下颌。

Open your mouth as wide as possible.

请尽可能张大嘴。

Bite down，please.

请咬合。

Please relax your tongue.

请放松舌头。

Rinse your mouth，please.

请漱口。

When did the tooth start to hurt?

这颗牙是什么时候开始疼的?

What kind of pain did you feel?

您感觉它是怎样的疼痛?

Did it hurt when I used the drill?

当我使用牙钻时您感觉疼吗?

I'll put some medical on the surface of your gums.

我将在您的牙龈表面涂些药物。

I will apply a topical anesthetic to numb the surface of the gum.

我将用表面麻醉药来麻醉您的牙龈。

Topic anesthetic will lessen the discomfort of the injection.

表面麻醉药将减轻注射的疼痛。

Are your lips and tongue numb?

您的嘴唇和舌头麻了吗？

The anesthetic will take effect in about three minutes.

三分钟左右麻醉药就会起效。

The numb feeling will continue for two or three hours.

麻木的感觉会持续两三个小时。

Please eat food after the numb feeling is gone.

等到麻木感觉消失后再进食。

The aspirator will remove the saliva from your mouth.

吸痰器会吸出您口腔里的唾液。

If you feel pain, please raise your hand.

如果感觉到疼痛，请举手。

Drilling may hurt you a little bit.

钻牙可能会使您感觉有点疼痛。

Don't be nervous if there is some swelling for a few days.

肿胀会持续两三天，请不要紧张。

If you have any problems of bleeding and severe pain, please tell us immediately.

如果出现出血和严重的疼痛，请立即告诉我们。

Don't rinse for 24 hours as it may affect blood coagulation.

24 小时内不要漱口，避免影响止血。

A small amount of blood in your mouth is normal until tomorrow.

直到明天，口腔里有少量血液都是正常的。

When you are not wearing your denture, be sure to keep them in a glass of water to keep wet.

当您不佩戴义齿时，请将它轻放在清水里，防止义齿变干。

There is possibility that the nerve will die in the future.

以后有神经坏死的可能。

The orthodontic treatment will improve not only the esthetic problems but also the function of the teeth.

正畸治疗不仅可以改善容貌还可以改善牙齿的功能。

(4) neurosurgery
神经外科

He is going to have a small bone window craniotomy.

他做的是小骨窗开颅术。

It is a better way to deal with the hypertensive intracranial hemorrhage.

这是处理高血压颅内出血的好方法。

Minimally invasive drainage is more effective than craniotomy for treating patients with cerebral hemorrhage in basal ganglia.

微创钻孔引流比开颅手术在治疗基底核部位脑出血方面更有效。

Pituitary tumor is a common deep tumor in the brain.

垂体瘤是一种常见的脑深部肿瘤。

During a craniotomy, a small section of the skull is cut away to allow the surgeon to gain access to the cause of the bleeding.

开颅手术中，颅骨会被切去一小部分，以便外科医生查出颅内出血的原因。

Following a craniotomy, you may have to be placed on a ventilator.

做完开颅手术，您可能会用到呼吸机。

A tumor can be described as benign or malignant.

肿瘤有良性的和恶性的。

No one knows the reason.

没人知道原因。

How about the patient's breath?

病人呼吸怎么样？

How about the patient's blood pressure?

病人血压怎么样？

How about the patient's oxygen saturation?

病人氧饱和度怎么样？

All is OK.

一切都挺好。

How much is urine volume?

尿量有多少？

What's the color of the urine?

尿颜色如何？

The urine bag is full, and change it please.

尿袋已满，请更换。

Please reduce blood pressure to 100/70.

请将血压降到 100/70。

The patient is moving lightly, and please deepen anesthesia.

患者正在微微动，请加深麻醉。

Is the cranial drill ready?

颅骨电钻准备好了吗？

The wire saw is broken, and please change it.

线锯断了，请更换一个。

Aneurysm has ruptured.

动脉瘤已经破了。

Give me aneurysm clamp, please.

请给我动脉瘤夹钳。

Please prepare clips of XXX.

请准备 XXX 牌动脉瘤夹。

Temporary aneurysm clip, please.

请给我临时动脉瘤夹。

Bipolar coagulation forceps, micro scissors, tumor forceps, please.

双极电凝镊,显微剪刀,肿瘤镊。

Small round pin threads X-suture.

小圆针穿 X 号线。

One more stitch.

再来一针。

Another pack of brain cotton pieces.

再来一包脑棉片。

We will begin to close the skull.

我们将关颅了。

(Give me)hydrogen peroxide and iodine.

请给我双氧水和活力碘。

Please protect his eyes with the incise drape.

请用切口膜保护他的眼睛。

Incline his head to the left side.

请将他的头偏向左侧。

(Give me a)bandage.

给我一个绷带。

Let us do the counting of all the instruments,gauze and others.

我们一起来清点手术器械、纱布和其他物品吧。

（5）general surgery

普外科

We will perform an appendectomy.

我们要做阑尾切除手术。

You should divide these lymph nodes into different groups.

您需要将这些淋巴结分组。

We need more warm saline for abdominal irrigation.

我们需要更多温热的生理盐水来冲洗腹腔。

It needs two tubes for abdominal drainage.

需要两根管子做腹腔引流。

Be careful of that vessel，it is a main artery.

小心那根血管，那是大动脉。

We can do it slowly.

我们可以慢慢做。

If you cannot deal with it，please tell your superior doctor.

如果您处理不了时，请告知您的上级医生。

Please call the head nurse quickly，we need help.

请赶快给护士长打电话，我们需要支援。

Please prepare the defibrillator.

请准备除颤仪。

（Give me an）abdominal retractor.

给我一个腹部拉钩。

Add chemotherapy medicine to water for abdominal irrigation.

将化疗药溶于水中冲洗腹腔。

Take out the clot and prevent it from bleeding.

取出凝血块并止血。

Suture and knot-tying is an important basic task for a surgical procedure.

缝合打结是外科手术重要的基本操作。

Clean the ultrasound scalpel please.

请将超声刀擦拭干净。

There is a chance to retain the obstructive small intestine and give more hot water to speed up its blood circulation.

这些梗阻的小肠还有挽救的机会，请给我更多的热水来加速它的血液循环。

Complete hepatic vascular occlusion can improve the safety of hepatectomy.

全肝血流阻断可提高切肝手术的安全性。

The patient's neck isn't exposed well, which will not be conductive to the operation.

患者的颈部没有暴露好，不利于手术操作。

This is the central lymph node.

这是中央组淋巴结。

This is 7th group of lymph node.

这是第 7 组淋巴结。

Give me a specimen tray.

请给我一个标本盘。

This is left/right pelvic lymph node.

这是左/右盆腔淋巴结。

This is left/right periaortic lymph node.

这是左/右腹主动脉旁淋巴结。

All lymph node specimens are placed separately.

所有淋巴结标本分开放置。

Her hand needs to be suspended to clean the axillary lymph nodes.

患者的手需要悬吊起来，方便清扫腋下淋巴结。

We are going to do the lymph node biopsy.

我们需要进行淋巴结活检手术。

Which side does he operate on, right or left?

他是做哪一侧手术，右边还是左边？

The result of rapid pathological examination is out.

快速病检结果出来了。

It's benign.

它是良性病变。

Only the left thyroid gland was removed.

患者只切除左侧甲状腺。

The spleen also needs to be removed and we should talk to her family.

她的脾脏也需要切除，我们需要和她家属谈谈。

Invite his family to the intraoperative room.

请他的家属来到术中谈话室。

The cancer has metastasized.

癌症已经转移了。

We still need to remove the inflammatory appendix.

我们还要切除发炎的阑尾。

We're ready to close the abdominal cavity.

我们准备关闭腹腔了。

Please start counting all sterilized instruments. gauze. cotton pads and so on.

请开始清点器械、纱布、棉垫等所有物品。

Give me the pastes.

给我几个敷贴。

It needs compression bandage.

需要加压包扎。

What is the name of the operation?

手术名称是什么?

The name of the operation must be the same as the record of the operation.

手术名称必须与手术记录保持一致。

(6) urinary surgery
泌尿外科

The operation name is removal of part of the urinary bladder.

手术名称是膀胱部分切除。

His surgery is performed at right side.

他的手术做的是右边。

Prepare for the nephrectomy immediately.

马上进行肾切除术。

We need to do the ureterostomy.

我们需要进行输尿管吻合术。

The patient will be posed at lateral position later.

接下来要将患者调整至侧卧位。

Cancer is a disease in which abnormal cells grow in an uncontrolled way.

癌症是一种异常细胞以不可控制的方式生长的疾病。

Bladder cancer is one of the most common cancers for men.

膀胱癌是男性疾病中最常见的癌症之一。

We will do the urethroplasty for this little boy.

我们要为这个小男孩进行尿道成形术。

Testicular torsion is serious which must be removed.

睾丸扭转情况较严重，不得不切除。

We have to do the vas deferens anastomosis.

我们需要进行输精管吻合术。

We only need to preserve one artery and lymphatic vessels.

我们只需要保留一根动脉和淋巴管。

The patient's blood pressure is so high that the operation may have to be stopped.

患者血压太高了，手术估计不能如期进行了。

There is a huge cyst on the kidney.

肾脏上有一个巨大囊肿。

Urethral dilator is required for urethral stricture.

尿道有狭窄，需要尿道扩张器。

Give me a glove and rubber tube, and I'll make an air bag.

给我一个手套和一个橡皮管来做气囊。

There isn't enough space to operate, and we need pump more carbon dioxide into it.

操作空间还不够大，我们需要继续进气。

Ureteral calculi are too big, so ureterolithotomy is necessary.

输尿管结石太大了，因此必须进行输尿管切开取石术。

Has the ureter been injuried?

输尿管损伤了吗？

Give me a piece of gauze to stop the bleeding.

给我一块纱条压迫止血。

I need to inject some methylene blue stain into the spermaduct.

我需要向输精管里注射一点亚甲蓝染色剂。

（7）orthopaedics

骨科

The prone position is frequently used in lumbar discectomy.

俯卧位经常用于腰椎间盘切除术中。

We should pay attention to the complications of orthopedic surgery.

我们要注意骨科手术的并发症。

The intraoperative autologous transfusion has higher value for the patients who underwent scoliosis orthomorphia.

自体血回输在脊柱侧弯矫形术中具有很高的应用价值。

Did the patient receive any antibiotic before the surgery?

这位患者的预防性抗生素已经应用了吗？

Another group of antibiotics?

追加一组抗生素？

The surgery is long, and we should remove this tissue quickly.

手术时间比较长，我们要加快切除这块组织。

Be careful!

小心！

Let us rest for a while.

我们休息一会儿吧。

We maybe need another three hours to finish this surgery.

我们可能还需要三个小时才能完成手术。

After we use a plaster cast on your right elbow, you should keep an eye on the color of the fingers.

我们给您的右肘打上石膏后，您得注意观察指头的颜色。

The fourth and fifth segments of lumbar spine are first positioned under the C-arm machine.

首先在 C 臂机下定位出腰椎第四和第五节。

The patient had multiple fractures that required open reduction and internal fixation in several location.

患者有多处骨折,全部都要进行切开复位内固定术。

Join treplacement requires a rigorous aseptic procedure.

关节置换术需要严格的无菌操作。

After the prone position is set, we should check the patient's compression area to prevent pressure ulcers.

俯卧位摆放好后,我们需要检查患者受压处以防发生压疮。

Give me the nucleus pulposus clamp please.

请给我髓核钳。

Please prepare the skin graft knife.

请准备植皮刀。

The bone knife is too dull.

骨刀太钝了。

One lamina spreader please.

需要一个椎板撑开器。

Is the polymethylmethacrylate(PMMA) bone cement ready?

PMMA 骨水泥准备好了吗?

The meniscus is broken and must be repaired.

半月板已经破损了,必须要修复。

(8) gynaecology and obstetrics
妇产科

We need an injection of pituitrin to shrink the uterus.

我们需要注射垂体后叶素来收缩子宫。

An assistant is needed to lift the uterus.

需要一个助手来举宫。

Is the gauze roll ready?

纱布卷做好了吗？

Use the water ball to block the vaginal opening.

用水球堵住阴道口。

Hysteroscopic surgery should not take too long.

宫腔镜手术不能花太长时间。

Does it hurt here?

这里痛不痛？

We are ready to break the amniotic membrane.

我们准备破羊膜了。

Suction preparation.

吸引器准备。

Continue to press.

继续按压。

The baby's head is out.

宝宝头出来了。

Cut the umbilical cord down.

断脐带。

Congratulations! It's a girl.

恭喜您，是一个女孩。

Oxytocin has been injected into natural solution.

催产素已经加到静脉输液里了。

10 U more injections of oxytocin.

再来 10 U 催产素注射液。

The placenta is intact.

娩出的胎盘是完整的。

Uterine contractions are very poor and it continues bleeding.

子宫收缩状态不佳，一直在持续出血。

The placenta is given to the hospital to deal with.

胎盘交给院方处理。

The patient needed umbilical cord blood for tests.

该患者需要抽取脐血进行检查。

How is the baby?

新生儿情况怎么样?

The baby needs to be sent to the neonatology department for observation.

新生儿需要送至新生儿科进行观察。

Baby's information needs to be registered.

新生儿的信息需要登记。

Mrs. Li, look at your baby and I'll take her back to the ward in advance.

李太太,来看看您的宝宝,我要提前将她送回病房。

Please prepare a specimen tray to collect specimens.

请准备标本盘接取标本。

Please prepare vigorous iodine gauze to disinfect vagina.

请准备活力碘纱布消毒阴道。

Tissue forceps are fixed at 12 o'clock. Please mark them with sutures.

组织钳固定处为 12 点的位置,请用缝线标记。

Please prepare iodoform gauze and vaseline gauze for packing.

准备碘仿纱布和凡士林纱布填塞。

Please observe the color of urine in the urine bag.

请观察一下尿袋内尿液的颜色。

Intravesical instillation of bladder with methylene blue saline.

请用亚甲蓝盐水进行膀胱灌注。

Please stop urine irrigation.

请停止灌尿。

There was no methylene blue in pelvic cavity, bladder was intact.

盆腔内无亚甲蓝，膀胱完好。

Please give me a drainage bag. I need to change the urine bag.

请给我一个引流袋，我需要更换尿袋。

Please dilute pituitrin one to one for on-stage injection.

请一比一稀释垂体后叶素，台上注射用。

Pituitrin is injected. The anesthesiologist should pay attention to the observation of blood pressure.

在台上注射垂体后叶素后，请麻醉医生注意观察血压。

Please maintain 10 U oxytocin intravenous drip.

请维持10U催产素静脉滴注。

Give me the uterine cavity balloon, prepare for oppression hemostasis.

请上宫腔球囊，准备压迫止血。

Give me 1-0 absorbable suture to sew the vaginal stump, please.

请给我 1-0 可吸收缝线，缝阴道残端。

Give me 2-0 absorbable suture to sew the ovaries, please.

请给我 2-0 可吸收缝线，缝卵巢。

Here is a broken intestinal tube. Please give me 4-0 absorbable suture to repair it.

此处肠管有破损，请给我 4-0 可吸收缝线修补。

Give me the rotary cutter.

请给我旋切器。

Prepare to suspend the peritoneum.

准备悬吊腹膜。

Give me a vaginal hook.

给我阴道拉钩。

Put a piece of gauze in the vagina, Please note.

阴道填塞小纱布一块,请注意备注。

Give me a longer vaginal speculum, please.

请给我一个较长的窥阴器。

Give me a vascular retrector.

给我血管拉钩。

3. communication of endoscopic surgery
腔镜类手术的术中沟通

Please open the air supply switch, and we start to build a pneumoperitoneum.

打开气源开关,我们开始建立气腹。

Please give me a bigger troca.

请给我一个大一点的穿刺器。

We need to block this blood vessel with a hem-o-lok.

我们需要用血管夹阻断这根血管。

Give me the endoscopic vascular forcep to separate the vessel.

给我一把腔镜血管钳来分离血管。

We should use the ultrasonic scalpel to finish this surgery.

我们需要用超声刀来完成这台手术。

We can choose three operation holes.

我们可以选择三个操作孔。

The tissue adhesion of this patient is terrible, and we should separate them firstly.

这名患者的组织粘连很严重,我们应该先将它们分开。

Uniportal video-assisted thoracoscopic pulmonary lobectomy requires the effective cooperation of surgical nurses.

单孔胸腔镜下肺叶切除术需要手术护士高效的配合。

Please ventilate the lungs, and we need to check for air leakage.

请向肺内进行通气，我们检查一下是否漏气。

There is a leak here and we need to tie a knot.

这个部位有点漏气，我们需要打结处理。

Give me the knot pusher.

请给我推结器。

We should use electric coagulation hook to remove the tissue.

我们需要使用电凝钩来切除这些组织。

The fallopian tubes need to pass fluid to check whether it is unobstructed.

输卵管需要通液来检查是否通畅。

Open the water pump to flush the abdominal cavity.

打开水泵，冲洗腹腔。

Adjust the position of head low and feet high.

调整头低脚高位。

The patient's eyes need to be protected because they're not closed.

患者眼睛没有闭合，需要保护一下。

Give me a transitting tube, please.

请给我一个转换器。

A metal clip, please.

请给我一个金属夹。

I need an absorbable clip.

我需要一个可吸收夹。

Change a dissecting forcep, please.

请换一个分离钳。

Grasping forcep, please.

请给我一个抓钳。

We are ready to take the specimen out. Please give me a specimen bag.

我们准备取出标本了,请给一个标本袋。

We can stop carbon dioxide pneumoperitoneum.

可以停止气腹状态了。

You should protect the lens.

请保护好镜头。

六、Postoperative recovery and handover

术后苏醒与交接

1. anesthesia recovery
麻醉苏醒期

Are you awake?

您醒了吗?

He is awake and can be extubated.

患者醒了,可以拔管了。

Are you OK? The operation is over, it is successful.

您还好吗? 手术结束了,很成功。

The patient is a little agitated and please give him some sedative.

患者有些烦躁,请给予镇静剂。

We put his/your X ray in this bag.

我们把他的/您的 X 片放在这个袋子里。

Let me help you put on your clothes.

让我帮您把衣服穿上吧。

Signature on the operational list, please.

请在清点单上签字。

Please open your eyes, the operation is finished.

请您睁开眼睛,手术已经结束了。

Now we will take you to the recovery room.

现在我们送您去康复室。

Now the doctor will take you back to your ward.

148

现在医生送您回病房。

Have a good rest.

好好休息。

Be careful and don't move, please.

请小心一点,不要动。

Keep still to avoid falling down.

保持不动,以防坠床。

Follow the advice of your primary nurse in your ward which will help you recuperate early.

请遵守您的责任护士给出的建议,这会有助于您早日康复。

Any questions you may ask your duty nurse.

有任何问题都可以问您病房的责任护士。

We will be glad to offer you our help.

我们很乐意帮助您。

This is automatic patient control acesodyne(PCA)pump.

这是自控止痛泵。

It helps you relieve the pain.

它帮助您缓解疼痛。

If you feel pain, please press this button.

如果您感到疼痛,就请按这个键。

Hello, Mrs. Zhang, how are you feeling now?

您好,张太太,您现在感觉怎么样?

Your operation went well, no complications.

您的手术很成功,没有并发症。

Although you will feel thirsty, you can't drink water now.

您确实会感到口渴,但是现在您不能喝水。

You are in stable condition.

您现在情况稳定。

Cough if you want.

如果您想咳嗽就请咳嗽。

I will start to suck the sputum for you.

我准备开始为您吸痰。

Let's monitor the patient's vital signs for a second.

我们再观察一下患者的生命体征。

ECG monitoring can be removed.

心电监护可以取下来了。

Let's remove the patient to this bed together.

我们一起将患者搬运至这张床上。

Send him to the anesthesia recovery room.

把他送到麻醉苏醒室吧。

2. shift to the ward
与病房的交接

We can start the shift.

我们可以开始交班了。

Please keep this urine tube in place.

请避免尿管滑脱。

These are his X rays and clothes.

这是他的 X 光片和衣服。

The intravenous catheter is still in place and the infusion is smooth.

静脉留置针固定牢靠,输注通畅。

There are no pressure ulcers on his body.

患者无压伤发生。

The patient has a gauze inside the vagina to remind the doctor to remove it in time.

患者阴道内塞有一块纱布，提醒医生及时取出来。

The drainage tube should be properly placed.

引流管需要妥善放置。

These are the rest of his medicine.

这是他剩下的药。

He can't drink or eat for the next × hours.

接下来×小时内不要给他喂水和吃东西。

Don't let him fall asleep.

不要让他睡熟了。

There is skin flushing on the sacral region of this patent which can be discolored by pressure.

患者骶尾部有点压红，但是压之可褪色。

A blister is formed on the patient's arm due to the pressure.

由于术中压迫导致患者手臂上出现一条水泡。

Please pay more attention to his pressure sores and tell us if you have any questions.

请多观察他的压疮情况，有任何问题请告知我们。

3. shift of the instruments
术后器械的交接

Please recycle instruments right now.

请立即过来回收器械。

Let us count the instruments together.

我们一起来清点器械。

The instrument is broken, please change it.

这个器械已经坏了，请更换。

The instrument is easy to be broken and please protect it with a cover.

这个器械容易损坏,请用保护套好好保护。

Is the total number of instruments correct?

器械总数量是对的吗?

I have rinsed them.

我已经冲洗过了。

Don't forget to record and signature.

不要忘记登记与签名。

If you finish the operation, please call me to recycle the instruments.

如果您手术完了,请打电话叫我来回收器械。

It is important to track the instruments.

器械的追溯十分重要。

This instrument is out of date and please sterilize again.

这个器械已经过期,请重新消毒。

It is wet and we can't use it.

这个已经湿了,我们不能使用。

The instrument is still dirty and you should clean it again.

这个器械仍然很脏,请重新清洗。

It is still in sterilization and we need to wait.

它仍在消毒中,我们还需要等待。

This instrument needs urgent treatment.

这个器械需要加急处理。

It will take several minutes for the instrument to be sterilized.

这个器械还需要几分钟才能消毒完毕。

The instrument failed to be sterilized and needs to be sterilized again.

器械消毒失败，需要重新消毒。

I need a gastrointestinal instrument set. Please send it to the operating room.

我需要一个胃肠器械包，请帮我送到手术间。

Ophthalmic instruments are all delicate, so please clean them carefully.

眼科器械均比较精细，请小心清洗。

How long will it take for urgent sterilization at high temperature?

紧急高温灭菌需要多长时间？

How long will it take to sterilize at low temperature at the fastest rate?

低温灭菌最快需要多久？

The patient has hepatitis C and the surgical instruments require special treatment.

患者有丙肝，使用过的器械需要特殊处理。

The surgical instruments have been sealed in double yellow trash bags.

手术器械已经用双层黄色垃圾袋密封起来。

六、术后苏醒与交接

七、Postoperative return visit
术后回访

Hello，××，I am a nurse from operating room，my name is...

您好，××，我是手术室护士，我的名字叫……

Do you remember me?

您还记得我吗？

I come to visit you.

我来看望您。

How are you feeling today?

您今天感觉如何？

Are you feeling better?

您感觉好些了吗？

Did you sleep well?

您睡得好吗？

Is there anything else that worries you?

您还有哪些不舒服的吗？

Did you pass gas?

您肠道通气了没有？

Have you been farting?

您肠道通气了吗？

Are you feeling comfortable?

您觉得舒服吗？

Do you feel pain?

您觉得痛吗？

Is your wound OK?

您的伤口还好吗？

Has the dressing of wound been changed?

伤口敷料换过了吗？

You should still keep the urine catheter.

您仍然需要保留着尿管。

Do you adapt to it?

您适应它了吗？

It will be removed soon.

它很快就会被拔掉。

Before removed, you will go through the bladder training.

在拔除之前，您需要进行膀胱训练。

You look well today.

您今天看起来气色很好。

As soon as your bowels are moving again, you can start to eat.

一旦您的肠管开始恢复蠕动，您就可以吃东西了。

Let's move on to talk about a few tips for safe swallowing which I'd like to go through with you. Is that OK?

咱们接着谈谈安全进食的相关事项，可以吗？

How about your appetite?

您食欲如何？

Does your stomach feel stuffed?

您感觉胃胀吗？

Do you feel nauseated?

您感觉恶心吗？

You cannot eat cold food.

您不能吃冷的食物。

Avoid eating greasy food.

不要吃油腻的食物。

You can continue with the pureed diet and thickened fluids until your swallow reflex is better.

在吞咽情况变好之前，请您坚持吃浓稠些的流食和纯膳食。

It's really important to avoid rush eating.

千万注意不要吃太快。

Take your time eating your food.

吃饭的时候需要细嚼慢咽。

Eat small amount of food several times a day.

每日少食多餐。

It's better to eat smaller meal than larger meal.

分批少吃比一次性多吃要好一些。

Don't drink and eat at the same time.

吃饭和喝水不要同时进行。

Try to avoid talking while eating.

吃饭的时候不要说话。

Relax and enjoy your meal.

吃饭的时候要放松。

After your meal, it's a good idea to sit up for around $\times$ minutes to let your food digest.

吃完饭后，最好是静坐×分钟让食物消化。

You must choose a proper diet：low fat，low salt，low sugar and low calorie intake，and eat more fruits and vegetables.

您必须科学饮食：低脂肪、低盐、低糖、低热量摄入，多吃水果和蔬菜。

You should have light food，a lot of vegetables and fruits.

您的饮食要清淡，多吃蔬菜和水果。

Have regular meals, keep a diet with a lot of vegetables, fruits and little meat.

饮食要规律,多吃蔬菜、水果,少吃肉类。

Too much salt will hurt your kidney, so you need to be careful about having salt or sodium.

过多的盐会伤肾,因此您吃含盐或含钠的食物必须小心。

You'd better stay away from alcohol and give up smoking.

您最好少碰烟酒。

Keep off alcohol and greasy food.

别喝酒,别吃油腻的食物。

I've brought a pain eveluating chart so you can explain your pain exactly.

我带来了病痛评估表帮您详细地描述您的疼痛级别。

Can you tell me on the scale of 0 to 10 what is the worst pain you've had in the last 24 hours in each area?

您能用 0~10 的评分来评价一下在过去 24 小时内每一处部位的疼痛程度吗?

Can you show me the first one on the picture of the body?

您能从这张全身图上指出第一处疼痛的部位吗?

What's the pain in your shoulder like?

肩膀处是怎样疼痛的?

When will the pain appear?

什么时候会出现这种疼痛?

What helps to relief the pain?

这种疼痛是如何缓解的呢?

Do you want to go to the toilet first?

您需要先去一下卫生间吗?

I'll just get your walking frame for you.

我来帮您取助行器。

If the wound does not hurt, you can get out of bed and work around.

如果伤口不那么疼,您可以下床活动。

That will help peristalsis of the intestine, which means you will pass gas a bit more easily and the distension will go away.

这样有助于恢复肠道蠕动,使气体排出减轻腹胀。

It's important to mobilize as soon as possible after your operation.

手术后及时活动很重要。

Swing your legs over the side of the bed slowly.

现在把您的双腿慢慢滑到床边。

Put your feet firmly on the floor.

把脚放稳到地上。

You're doing very well. Now, take a few steps.

您做得很好。现在走几步试试。

Just go for a short walk today. Tomorrow you can go a little bit further.

今天走一小段就行,明天您可以多走点。

You should sit up that can help you breath deeper and cough out phlegm more smoothing, and prevent pneumonia.

您应该坐起来,这样可以帮助您深呼吸,使痰较容易咳出,并防止肺炎。

Sit on the edge of the bed, and if you don't feel dizzy you can get out of bed.

您先在床边坐坐,没有感到头晕就可以下床了。

If you feel dizzy, you can't go out of bed.

如果您觉得头晕,就不能下床。

Please turn from side to side every two or three hours.

请您每两三个小时翻一次身。

You can try walking around the room or corridor.

您可以试着在房间或走廊里走走。

Can you answer me some questions?

您能回答我一些问题吗？

How do you think of our preoperative nursing?

您觉得我们手术室术前护理如何？

Did they give you any help mentally?

她们在心理上给予您帮助吗？

Can you give us some suggestions?

您能给我们一些意见吗？

What do you think that we need to improve?

您认为我们在哪些方面还需要改进？

Are you satisfied with the nurse's attitude?

您对护士的态度满意吗？

Are you satisfied with the nurses' service?

您对我们的护理服务还满意吗？

Is there anything that constantly upsets you?

还有什么困扰您的事吗？

The operation is very successful.

手术很成功。

You will be prescribed medication for pain relief, please tell one of the nurses when you are in pain.

当您疼痛时请告诉护士，医生会给您开止痛药。

I don't know when you can discharge.

我不知道您什么时候可以出院。

It depends on your recovery.

取决于您的恢复情况。

You have to stay here for another one week.

您还得住一个星期的院。

You are going to be discharged the day after tomorrow.

您后天就可以出院了。

You can go home in about a week.

大约一个星期您就可以出院了。

After you are released from the hospital, you will need to stay at home and have a good rest for the first week.

您出院后,第一周还需要待在家里,好好地休息。

If you feel worse, please come back to the hospital right away.

如果您觉得病重了,请马上来医院。

I suggest you walk around and do some light exercises.

我建议您在地上走走,做些轻微的锻炼。

I'm glad to see you are recovering so well.

我很高兴看到您恢复得如此好。

It won't take long to recover.

很快您就可以康复了。

You will have to rest when you go home, just gentle exercise at first and do not lift anything heavy for a few weeks.

您回家后需要好好休息,在几个星期内可以做一些轻微的运动,但不要提重的东西。

It will take you at least one month's rest to recover completely.

您至少需要休息一个月才会完全恢复。

You must avoid mental stress and tiring work from now on.

从现在起,您必须避免精神紧张和太累的工作。

Keep a mood relaxed is essential to health.

保持心情舒畅，这是保证健康的最基本条件。

If you want to maintain a good level of health, you must have the right lifestyle.

如果您想保持良好的健康水平，就必须有正确的生活方式。

Exercising more everyday, because bones usually grow stronger when they bear more weight.

平时应该多锻炼身体，骨骼承受压力后才能变结实。

You may take a walk, shadowbox, or ride bicycle, etc.

您可以散步、打拳、骑车，等等。

Try to maintain a half-an-hour to one-hour walk everyday.

坚持每天散步 0.5～1 小时。

For a speedy recovery, you have to endure the difficulty for now.

忍耐暂时的痛苦，争取最快、最好的康复。

You should keep taking your medicine, and continue cooperate with us on your diet, daily activities, and self-monitoring.

希望您回家后能坚持服药，并在饮食、日常活动及自我检测等方面与我们配合。

You should pay attention to regulating your life such as getting up and going to bed regularly and not drinking or smoking too much.

您要注意的是规律生活，如定时起床、定时睡觉，不要过多地饮酒和抽烟。

Please be careful and never stop medication or take other medicines by yourself.

请您一定不要随便服药与停药。

You will also need to monitor your body temperature, blood pressure, urine quantity by yourself.

您需要自己学会监测体温、血压、尿量。

After six months you can resume to full-time work, gradually from light work to normal work.

术后六个月,您可以恢复工作,由轻松一点的工作逐步过渡到正常工作。

If you need any more information, come and see me.

如果您需要了解更多的情况,请来找我。

There is no sex for the next three months.

接下来三个月不能同房。

Take medicine regularly every day.

每天定时吃药。

Monitor the date of ovulation each mouth.

监测每个月的排卵日期。

You still have a chance to get pregnant again.

您还有机会怀孕。

Take good care of yourself.

请您多保重。

You will be all right soon.

您很快就会好起来的。

You must feel confident that you can overcome the disease.

您必须要树立战胜疾病的信心。

Please go to the hospital regularly for reexamination.

请定期到医院进行复查。

八、CPR and defibrillation
CPR 与除颤

Put the person on his or her back on a firm surface.

将病人放置于一块硬板上。

Kneel next to the person's neck and shoulders.

跪于病人颈肩旁。

Place the heel of one hand over the center of the person's chest, between the nipples. Place anther hand on top of the first hand.

一只手掌根放于胸正中两乳头连线中点，另一只手放于第一只手上。

Keep your elbows straight and position your shoulders directly above your hands.

双肘伸直，肩部在手掌之上。

Use your upper body weight (not just your arms) as you push straight down on (compress) the chest 1/2 to 2 inches.

保持腰背挺直，使用上半身垂直力量按压胸腔，按压深度大致为 1/2～2 英寸。

Press hard and fast—give two compressions per second, or about 110 compressions per minute at least.

用力快速地按压，每秒 2 次或者至少每分钟 110 次。

After 30 compressions, remove the oral secretion with head to one side.

按压 30 次以后，头偏向一侧，清除口腔分泌物。

Open the person' airway. Put your palm on the person 's forehead and gently push down.

打开患者气道，一手放在前额轻轻向下压。

Then with another hand with EC method, gently lift the chin forward to open the airway, and supply oxygen with the flow of 10 L/min.

另一只手用 EC 法氧气罩给氧,轻抬下颌开放气道,提供每分钟 10 升的氧气吸入。

Prepare to give two rescue breaths. Give the first rescue breath—lasting one second—and watch to see if the chest rises.

准备两次人工呼吸,第一次完毕后停歇一秒并观察胸廓是否有起伏。

If it does rise, give the second breath. If the chest doesn't rise, repeat the head tilt-chin lift and then give the second breath.

如果胸廓有起伏,进行第二次呼吸;如果胸廓没有起伏,重复抬头仰额再继续给氧。

Begin chest compressions—go to "circulation" below.

开始胸外按压,按循环继续操作。

Continue CPR until there are signs of movement.

持续进行 CPR 直至患者有苏醒活动体征。

Assess the situation before starting CPR.

开始 CPR 之前首先要评估者。

Please switch it on.

请打开开关。

Press the charge button.

请按充电按钮。

Select the nonsynchronous biphasic wave 120J(joule).

选择非同步双向波 120 焦。

Attention! Everyone Clear!

注意! 所有人退后!

Discharge! Is that OK?

放电！好了吗？

I'll administer epinephrine to him.

我要给他用肾上腺素。

Hurry up!

快点！

The patient's heartbeat has recovered.

患者心跳已经恢复。

As an important emergency device, defibrillator-monitor has played an irreplaceable role in rescuing a heart attack patient.

除颤监护仪作为一种重要的急救设备，在心脏病患者突发事件的抢救过程中具有不可替代的作用。

It is very important to save serious patients.

(除颤)对于挽救危重病人的生命有着重要的意义。

八、CPR与除颤

参 考 文 献

[1] 刘锴. 新编实用护士英语[M]. 沈阳：辽出临图字出版社，1993.187.

[2] 郑一宁，吴欣娟，杨潇. 护理英语会话[M]. 北京：人民军医出版社，2010.112.

[3] 王文秀，冯永平. 医务英语会话[M]. 2版. 北京：人民卫生出版社，2001.692.

[4] Linda. C. Adam. 实用医学英语会话（护士篇）[M]. 肖幸锐，译. 北京：中国水利水电出版社，2008. 210.

[5] 戴九龙，高蕾. 现代医院英语情景会话[M]. 北京：军事医学科学出版社，2007.412.

[6] 洪津. 实用护理英语情境口语[M]. 天津：天津大学出版社，2010.165.

[7] 余立江. 口腔临床英语[M]. 北京：中国协和医科大学出版社，2007.144.

[8] 强丽宁，杨潇. 护理英语[M]. 北京：人民军医出版社，2014.226.

[9] 李定钧. 医学英语词汇学[M]. 上海：复旦大学出版社，2006.502.

[10] 唐巧英. 医护英语[M]. 北京：外语教学与研究出版社，2015.106.

[11] 倪晓红. 医学英语情景实用指南[M]. 北京：世界图书出版公司，2013.208.

[12] 王文秀，王颖，贾轶群. 英汉对照医务英语会话[M]. 3版. 北京：人民卫生出版社，2016.800.

[13] 徐红莉，杨桂荣. 涉外护理英语[M]. 北京：对外经贸大学出版社，2013.217.

实用手术室专业英语会话

[14]　王洵.实用护理英语［M］.南京:南京大学出版社,
　　　2011.212.

[15]　何国平,曾颖,冯辉.护理专业英语［M］.中南大学出版
　　　社,2011.301.

参　考　文　献